Pharmacoinvasive Therapy in Acute Myocardial Infarction

Fundamental and Clinical Cardiology

Editor-in-Chief
Samuel Z. Goldhaber, M.D.
Harvard Medical School
and Brigham and Women's Hospital
Boston, Massachusetts

Pharmacoinvasive Therapy in
Acute Myocardial Infarction

edited by
Harold Dauerman

Fletcher Allen Health Care,
Burlington, Vermont, U.S.A.
University of Vermont,
Burlington, U.S.A.

Burton E. Sobel

Fletcher Allen Health Care,
Burlington, Vermont, U.S.A.
University of Vermont,
Burlington, U.S.A.

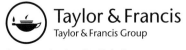

Taylor & Francis
Taylor & Francis Group

Boca Raton   London   New York   Singapore

Although great care has been taken to provide accurate and current information, neither the author(s) nor the publisher, nor anyone else associated with this publication, shall be liable for any loss, damage, or liability directly or indirectly caused or alleged to be caused by this book. The material contained herein is not intended to provide specific advice or recommendations for any specific situation.

Trademark notice: Product or corporate names may be trademarks or registered trademarks and are used only for identification and explanation without intent to infringe.

Library of Congress Cataloging-in-Publication Data

Pharmacoinvasive therapy in acute myocardial infarction / edited by Harold L. Dauerman and Burton E. Sobel.
    p. ; cm. -- (Fundamental and clinical cardiology)
  Includes bibliographical references and index.
  ISBN 0-8247-5940-0
    1. Myocardial infarction--Chemotherapy. 2. Transluminal angioplasty. I. Dauerman, Harold L. II. Sobel, Burton E. III. Series.
    [DNLM: 1. Myocardial Infarction--therapy. 2. Angioplasty, Transluminal, Percutaneous Coronary. 3. Combined Modality Therapy. 4. Thrombolytic Therapy. WG 300 P536 2005]
  RC685.I6P48 2005
  616.1'237061--dc22

                                 2004063456

ISBN: 0-8247-5940-0

This book is printed on acid-free paper.

Headquarters
Marcel Dekker, 270 Madison Avenue, New York, NY 10016, U.S.A.
tel: 212-696-9000; fax: 212-685-4540

World Wide Web
http://www.dekker.com

Series Introduction

Marcel Dekker, Inc., has focused on the development of various series of beautifully produced books in different branches of medicine. These series have facilitated the integration of rapidly advancing information for both the clinical specialist and the researcher.

My goal as editor-in-chief of the Fundamental and Clinical Cardiology series is to assemble the talents of world-renowned authorities to discuss virtually every area of cardiovascular medicine. In the current monograph, Drs. Harold L. Dauerman and Burton E. Sobel have edited a much-needed and timely book. Future contributions to this series will include books on molecular biology, interventional cardiology, and clinical management of such problems as coronary artery disease and ventricular arrhythmias.

Samuel Z. Goldhaber

Preface

Coronary thrombolysis and primary infarct percutaneous coronary intervention (PCI) in the treatment of ST segment elevation myocardial infarction (STEMI) are conventionally viewed as mutually exclusive alternative therapeutic modalities. However, well established principles and a great deal of recently acquired information support the view that the two in combination are synergistic. We shall refer to the combination as "pharmacoinvasive therapy." This terminology emphasizes the notion of synergy and is more descriptively accurate than the often used "facilitated angioplasty." The focus of this book is the conceptual basis underlying pharmacoinvasive therapy and the history of its refinement in the treatment of patients with acute ST segment elevation myocardial infarction.

The development of pharmacoinvasive therapy has not been straightforward. In fact, current clinical research in this area reflects a renaissance of interest in the combined therapeutic approach. Pioneering studies of pharmacologically induced recanalization by Chazov and Rentrop during the 1970s utilized an invasive approach to deliver intracoronary fibrinolytic drugs. Subsequently, intravenously administered fibrinolytic agents proved to be promising. The potential utility of intravenous administration of fibrinolytic agents coupled with prompt, subsequent mechanical recanalization (balloon angioplasty) was recognized and evaluated. However, a high incidence of complications and generally negative results led to a rejection of the use of the two approaches in combination. In addition, they led to the two treatment modalities becoming considered as being mutually exclusive alternatives.

Refinements and improvements in pharmacologic ("thrombolysis") and mechanical approaches ("primary angioplasty") to recanalization have been impressive. Randomized clinical trials and registries have been used to compare and contrast the two, but assessment of both in combination lay dormant until quite recently. Improvements in coronary thrombolysis and coronary interventions now make reassessment of pharmacoinvasive therapy particularly desirable. Reassessment is indicated given the inherent limitations, when used alone, in both pharmacologic (failure to restore flow adequately) and mechanical approaches (unavoidable delay that can prolong the time to initiation of reperfusion).

Section I of this book describes: 1) the conceptual basis underlying pharmacoinvasive therapy, 2) the efficacy and limitations of each of its two components when used alone, and 3) the reductions in mortality that have been accomplished with each. Section II addresses the failure of early trials to demonstrate the benefit of combinations of balloon angioplasty coupled with antecedent coronary thrombolysis.

The PACT trial was a reevaluation of a combined approach. It stimulated further reassessment of combination therapy with the use of registries and substudies in randomized clinical trials. These more recent studies are described in detail in a section devoted to the evolution of pharmacoinvasive therapy.

Subsequent material focuses on the rationale for several studies planned or already underway. These studies are designed to clarify the role of glycoprotein IIB/IIIa inhibitors, low molecular weight heparin, novel anticoagulants, and novel plasminogen activators in facilitating safe and effective initial pharmacologic recanalization while avoiding compromise of benefits that can be conferred by prompt, subsequent percutaneous coronary intervention (PCI).

The last section addresses the design of studies needed to delineate optimal treatment of specific patient populations with STEMI including those at highest risk. One such population is the elderly.

The book concludes with a chapter entitled "Controversy and Convergence." It summarizes the progressive nature of development of refinements in pharmacoinvasive therapy. The chapter emphasizes the underlying principles contributing to the rebirth of interest in this therapeutic modality.

This book was designed to trace the rebirth of pharmacoinvasive therapy attributable to the accomplishments, ingenuity, and diligence of numerous investigators who have been devoted to the care of patients with acute myocardial infarction. The editors are fortunate to have engaged several of these outstanding authorities in presenting their observations, interpretations, and insights.

Contributors

Elliott M. Antman   Brigham and Women's Hospital, Boston, Massachusetts, U.S.A.

Alan K. Berger   University of Minnesota, Minneapolis, Minnesota, U.S.A.

Azan S. Binbrek   Rashid Hospital, Dubai, U.A.E.

Eugene Braunwald   Brigham and Women's Hospital, Boston, Massachusetts, U.S.A.

Harold L. Dauerman   University of Vermont, Burlington, Vermont, U.S.A.

Simon R. Dixon   William Beaumont Hospital, Royal Oak, Michigan, U.S.A.

Matthew Gutierrez   University of Vermont, Burlington, Vermont, U.S.A.

Robert Harrington   Duke Clinical Research Institute, Durham, North Carolina, U.S.A.

Harlan M. Krumholz   Yale University School of Medicine and Yale–New Haven Hospital, New Haven, Connecticut, U.S.A.

David J. Moliterno   University of Kentucky, Lexington, Kentucky, U.S.A.

William W. O'Neill   William Beaumont Hospital, Royal Oak, Michigan, U.S.A.

Edward L. Portnay   Yale University School of Medicine, New Haven, Connecticut, U.S.A.

Nayan S. Rao   Rashid Hospital, Dubai, U.A.E.

Matthew Roe   Duke Clinical Research Institute, Durham, North Carolina, U.S.A.

Jacqueline Saw   Vancouver General Hospital, University of British Columbia, Vancouver, British Columbia, Canada

David J. Schneider   University of Vermont, Burlington, Vermont, U.S.A.

Kawar Singh   Duke Clinical Research Institute, Durham, North Carolina, U.S.A.

Burton E. Sobel   University of Vermont, Burlington, Vermont, U.S.A.

Alan J. Tiefenbrunn   Washington University of St. Louis, St. Louis, Missouri, U.S.A.

Contents

I

Approaches to Reperfusion in the Treatment of STEMI: Thrombolysis or Primary PCI

1

The Rationale Underlying Pharmacoinvasive Therapy

**BURTON E. SOBEL and
HAROLD L. DAUERMAN**
University of Vermont
Burlington, Vermont, U.S.A.

I. INTRODUCTION

A compelling question confronting clinicians is how to optimally treat acute ST segment elevation myocardial infarction (STEMI). Over the past several decades, it has become clear that early recanalization of the infarct-related artery (IRA) is pivotal. How to best achieve this objective remains hotly debated. Some argue that thrombolysis is the preferred modality. Others promulgate primary percutaneous coronary intervention (PCI). Some advocate a combination, conventionally denoted as facilitated PCI. However, thrombolysis does not literally facilitate PCI. It may, in fact, render it more difficult. Furthermore, the combination deserves to be denoted as a specific entity with attributes that may be synergistic. Thus, we shall refer to the combination as pharmacoinvasive therapy. To better understand the potential synergies of thrombolysis and acute infarct PCI, it is instructive to carefully consider the evolution of recanalization therapy itself.

Before the advent of coronary care units, hospital mortality associated with acute STEMI was approximately 30%. Physicians caring for afflicted patients could do little besides provide oxygen, ameliorate pain, and treat congestive heart failure. Prognosis was dichotomous. Survival or death was generally declared within 48 hours. As access to prompt defibrillation became common, the picture changed radically. Patients who survived were recognized as being members of a heterogeneous group. Some would experience late, recurrent fatal or nonfatal coronary events. Others would slowly deteriorate and ultimately develop cardiogenic shock leading to death. Some would make a "complete" recovery with return to work.

It was in this context that Dr. Eugene Braunwald formulated a novel perception of the syndrome of acute myocardial infarction (AMI). His hypothesis was that AMI is a dynamic process, the outcome of which is determined largely by the extent of infarction sustained (infarct size). Infarct size was hypothesized to be a consequence of the severity and persistence of an imbalance between myocardial oxygen supply and myocardial oxygen demand. One of the first experimental animal studies performed to test this then-revolutionary view concluded: "Of greatest interest, from the clinical point of view, is the finding that the severity and extent of myocardial ischemic injury resulting from coronary occlusion could be radically altered not only by pretreatment … but also by an appropriate intervention as late as 3 hours after the coronary occlusion" (1).

It took only a few years for investigators to establish a striking relationship between infarct size and hemodynamic consequences and to determine that prognosis was related to the extent of infarction sustained (2,3). Restoration of the balance between impaired myocardial oxygen supply and demand soon became a focus of research. Three approaches were contemplated: (a) reduction of myocardial oxygen demand through reduction of afterload among other measures, (b) increasing myocardial oxygen supply with pharmacological or mechanical recanalization (4), and (c) enhancing myocardial metabolism to induce cardiocyte protection (1). The evolution and extent of infarction were found to be modifiable by diminishing the intensity of determinants of myocardial oxygen requirements (5). In addition, augmentation of myocardial oxygen supply by coronary recanalization was shown to diminish the extent of myocardial necrosis (6). Unfortunately, however, potential synergies between modes of recanalization applied sequentially were not evaluated. Ultimately, thrombolysis and PCI became viewed as mutually exclusive alternatives.

II. THE IMPORTANCE OF RAPID RECANALIZATION

The dynamic nature of STEMI and the concept of limiting infarct size led to methods to recanalize occluded coronary arteries by pharmacological means (7–11). The outcomes of several large, early clinical trials were not impressive. One reason was that methods for determining infarct size were not yet available. The reliance upon mortality as an exclusive endpoint in some studies precluded recognition of the clinical efficacy of early coronary recanalization.

Chazov et al. (12) and Rentrop et al. (13) initially demonstrated that intracoronary fibrinolytic drugs could indeed initiate prompt recanalization with favorable effects on the heart and on the patient. Their work ushered in the utilization of coronary recanalization as a primary treatment for acute myocardial infarction. It soon became clear that the beneficial effects of coronary thrombolysis on the heart were highly dependent upon the rapidity of reperfusion (14–25). Coronary angioplasty was in its infancy. Although the potential utility of PCI performed after pharmacological activation of the fibrinolytic system was being explored, additive benefits were not observed (26–30). Unfortunately, it appeared that excessive complications compromised this pharmacoinvasive approach to treatment of STEMI. In the context of these negative developments, combined pharmacoinvasive approaches were largely abandoned.

III. RECOGNITION OF THE PRIMACY OF RAPIDITY OF THROMBOLYSIS IN REDUCING INFARCT SIZE

As we have noted previously (30), The Fibrinolytic Therapy Trialists' Collaborative Group summarized results from early clinical trials as follows: 35 lives could be saved per 1000 patients with STEMI when treatment was initiated within the first hour after onset of symptoms. By contrast, fewer (16 per 1000) lives could be saved when treatment had to be delayed for as long as 7–12 hours (8). American College of Cardiology/American Heart Association (ACC/AHA) AMI guidelines state that "the earlier therapy begins, the better the outcome, with the greatest benefit . . . when (thrombolytic) therapy is given in the first 3 hours" (9). Results of studies in experimental animals (14), the landmark GISSI 1 clinical trial (19), the MITI trial (31), and numerous other studies of recanalization (32–36) are consistent with the view that a major determinant of the efficacy of recanalization in reducing the extent of infarction is the rapidity of its implementation.

IV.   THE EMERGENCE OF PRIMARY PCI

Remarkable progress was made between 1975 and 1997 in reducing hospital mortality associated with STEMI (Fig. 1.1) (37), progress attributable largely to advances in pharmacological treatment. The use of primary PCI as the mode of recanalization did not become prominent until later (38). However, limitations of coronary thrombolysis were well recognized. For example, restoration of complete (TIMI grade 3) flow occurred in only 60% of patients treated with thrombolytic drugs (Fig. 1.2) (39–42). Because survival was found to be linked closely to induction of TIMI grade 3 flow (40), vigorous investigation of invasive methods to achieve more complete coronary recanalization was pursued (39–42).

Acute infarct artery PCI was demonstrated initially to be feasible in conjunction with intracoronary thrombolysis in a small registry study reported in 1982 (43). The approach evolved quickly to one in which the intracoronary thrombolysis component was abandoned. The separation of mechanical and pharmacological approaches was reinforced by results in a small (56-patient), but very influential, randomized trial comparing primary PCI with administration of intracoronary streptokinase in 1986 (44). Primary PCI led to greater recovery of left ventricular function. Results from another relatively small, randomized trial (n = 142) were concordant. They demonstrated greater recovery of left ventricular function with primary PCI compared with intravenous streptokinase (45). The Primary Angioplasty in Myocardial Infarction

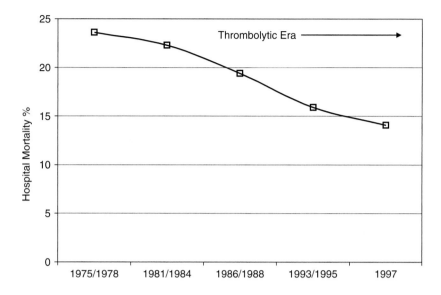

Figure 1.1 Improved survival in patients with STEMI in the 1975–1997 interval. The marked improvement reflects the impact of pharmacologically induced recanalization. (Adapted from Ref. 37.)

(PAMI) trial, a 395-patient randomized clinical trial, compared primary angioplasty with administration of tissue-type plasminogen activator (t-PA). It reported a remarkable difference in early mortality (from 6.5% to 2.6%; $p = 0.06$) favoring mechanical intervention. TIMI grade 3 flow was demonstrable in 90% of the patients who had been treated invasively (46). Nevertheless, the impact of this important trial on the care of patients with STEMI from 1993 to 1997 was relatively modest. Only 16% of patients with STEMI were being treated with primary angioplasty during this interval (38).

Important practical barriers have limited the widespread adoption of primary PCI for the treatment of STEMI. The fact that fewer than 25% of hospitals in the United States and fewer than 10% of hospitals in Europe have facilities for coronary angiography is a formidable factor (47,48). Several randomized, clinical trials designed to compare primary PCI with coronary thrombolysis for treatment of STEMI followed the

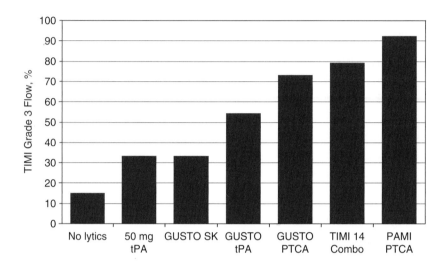

Figure 1.2 Achievement of normal and full coronary recanalization (TIMI Grade 3 flow) with multiple strategies. The most complete recanalization results from primary angioplasty as shown in the GUSTO IIB and PAMI trials. (From Refs. 39,41,46.)

PAMI trial. The GUSTO IIb substudy (Global Use of Strategies to Open Occluded Coronary Arteries) randomized 1138 patients with STEMI to t-PA or primary PCI and showed that the primary combined endpoint of death, nonfatal reinfarction, or stroke at 30 days was significantly reduced with primary PCI (9.6 compared with 13.7%; $p = 0.03$) (41). Somewhat surprisingly, however, the striking reduction in mortality seen in the PAMI trial was not confirmed (5.7 vs. 7.0%; $p = $ NS), probably in part because of differences in inclusion criteria. Thus, the GUSTO IIb substudy did not settle matters. Instead, it sparked further debate regarding the relative benefits of primary PCI in randomized clinical trials and in clinical practice. Analyses came to different conclusions: the registry results demonstrated no mortality benefit for primary PCI, whereas the trial results suggested a consistent reduction of mortality (49–51).

This divergence appears to be attributable in part to differences in patient populations in randomized trials compared with those in registries (52). Additional factors include the influence of performance

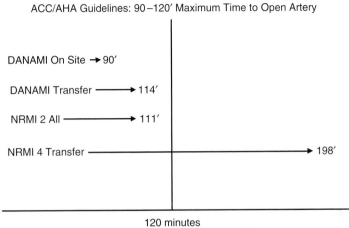

ACC/AHA Guidelines: 90–120′ Maximum Time to Open Artery

DANAMI On Site → 90′

DANAMI Transfer ——→ 114′

NRMI 2 All ——→ 111′

NRMI 4 Transfer ————————————→ 198′

120 minutes
Median Time from Hospital Presentation to Open Artery

Figure 1.3 A contrast between the induction of rapid recanalization in clinical practice with primary PCI (National Registry of Myocardial Infarction, NRMI) compared with results in recent randomized clinical trials of Primary PCI (DANAMI-2). The median time to coronary opening for on-site and transfer patients is substantially less in the trial compared with that seen in clinical practice, particularly when transfer is required. (From Refs. 59,60,71.)

of lower volumes of PCI by operators and institutions in registries as well as delay in time to treatment with PCI in clinical practice (53–55). Although more primary PCI randomized trials have been performed recently (56–58), their results have not resolved the underlying issues that continue to limit widespread adoption of primary PCI. Thus, the impressive reduction in reinfarction with primary PCI compared with t-PA in DANAMI 2 reflects experience in highly selected centers acting in a coordinated fashion that is not necessarily indicative of clinical practice in general. The median door-to-balloon times in the DANAMI 2 population for both on-site and transported patients (<110 min) (58) does not reflect clinical experience in the United States (59,60) (Fig. 1.3). Thus, a question persists: Can the apparent superiority of primary PCI in randomized trials be extrapolated to clinical practice such that thrombolysis for treatment of STEMI should be abandoned? We believe that an alternative, more helpful question is: Can the benefits of primary PCI be augmented by antecedent coronary thrombolysis providing a unified pharmacoinvasive approach in the treatment of all patients with STEMI?

V. PRINCIPLES SUPPORTING THE COMBINED USE OF THROMBOLYSIS AND PCI

The need to compare strategies such as pharmacological coronary thrombolysis and primary PCI led to refinement of endpoints used in studies of patients with STEMI. Many endpoints were developed for the assessment of these approaches, including those delineating the rapidity and persistence of coronary artery recanalization, the impact of intervention on the extent of infarction and ventricular function, and the impact on myocardial perfusion (61). Several lessons were learned. The efficacy of coronary thrombolysis was determined by the extent to which ongoing coagulation could be suppressed and fibrinolysis enhanced without precipitating bleeding (62) as well as by the rapidity of its initiation, in part because fresh clots lyse much more rapidly than established ones (63). The magnitude of restoration of flow (as measured by TIMI flow grade) and its persistence were found to be powerful determinants of prognosis (39,42). Avoidance of early reocclusion and maintenance of functional integrity of the microcirculation were shown to be critical determinants of an effective outcome (61,64,65). The incidence of bleeding was affected by the choice of specific combinations of conjunctive drugs used to induce reperfusion (fibrinolytic agents, anticoagulants, antiplatelet agents) (65–67).

Regardless of the nature of the endpoint used, the rapidity of coronary reperfusion was found to be of paramount importance (14,19,32–36,67–69). As much as 80% of the potential benefit conferred by coronary reperfusion via thrombolysis was found to be lost when reperfusion was delayed for as little as 3 hours following the onset of ischemic injury (32). Although some controversy exists with respect to the influence of early reperfusion on mortality after primary PCI (33,69), data from both multicenter trials and registries are consistent with increased mortality associated with delays in initiation of primary PCI (Fig. 1.4) (34–36,53).

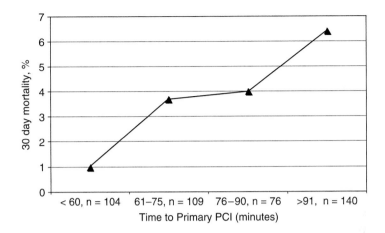

Figure 1.4   The importance of time to reperfusion for patients with STEMI is a unifying principal of treatment with primary PCI, thrombolytic therapy, or both. Results in GUSTO IIb trial demonstrate an increase in mortality as a function of delay in door to time of primary PCI. (From Ref. 34.)

The importance of time to reperfusion in patients with STEMI treated with primary PCI compared with thrombolytic drugs has recently been reexamined with respect to the extent of myocardial salvage (70). This study illustrates an ongoing difficulty in correlating outcomes with respect to time from symptom onset to balloon inflation as opposed to the interval from hospital admission to balloon inflation. Determination of the former is confounded by variability in the relationship between symptom onset and onset of irreversible ischemic injury as well as inaccuracies in reporting times of symptom onset. The relationship between time from hospital presentation to time to recanalization with primary PCI is clearer (34,53).

VI.   WHAT HAVE WE LEARNED THAT IS FUNDAMENTAL?

Three cardinal principles apply to the use of thrombolysis, PCI, or the two in combination for recanalization of an occluded infarct-related artery:

- Rapidity of reperfusion is a major determinant of improved survival in patients with STEMI.
- The magnitude of flow through the artery harboring the culprit lesion is a major determinant of improved survival.
- Two serious complications can occur with either modality — bleeding and reinfarction. Their frequency in specific patient populations influences the relative efficacy of either approach.

These principles and careful analysis of study design are necessary for optimal interpretation and application of results in clinical trials to clinical practice.

VII.   RECANALIZATION FOR TREATMENT OF STEMI

Debate has focused too long on the question of the relative value of primary PCI compared with thrombolysis (49). Protagonists of each buttressed their positions with reference to advances in pharmacological regimens [combined therapy with GP IIb/IIIa inhibitors (65,66,68)] and advances in technology [use of stents (56)]. In fact, the debate persisted because of a flawed, historically based presumption: "Routine, immediate angioplasty does not provide an improved outcome after thrombolytic [drug] administration" (25,71,72). Thus, the cardiology community has been driven toward an either/or approach.

The flawed presumption is predicated, in part, on early experience. The separation of early PCI from thrombolytic therapy was based on the observed lack of superiority and high incidence of adverse events in early trials of thrombolysis in which immediate PCI was being assessed (26–29). However, this adverse experience must be reexamined in the light of recent results from registries and later trials (72–77). Adverse event rates have been reduced with the use of either half-dose or clot-selective fibrinolytic agents, conjunctive anticoagulant and antiplatelet therapy, and advances in PCI technology (stenting). Thus, although a prohibition against early PCI after thrombolysis was supported by data from the important trials of thrombolysis in the 1980s, more recent information is not necessarily concordant.

A striking example can be seen in the results in the Plasminogen Activator Angioplasty Compatibility Trial (PACT). In this study patients with STEMI were randomized to treatment with half-dose t-PA (50 mg) compared with placebo. All patients underwent early PTCA. Immediate thrombolysis doubled the incidence of TIMI grade 3 flow (from 15 to 33%) at the time of initial angiography. A similar phenomenon was observed recently in the GRACIA II study reported at the 25th European Society of Cardiology Congress in Vienna. Antecedent thrombolysis preserved the benefits of PCI when it was performed within 3 hours. In PACT, left ventricular function was preserved in those with TIMI grade 3 flow at the time of initial angiography. In contradistinction to the results of trials of thrombolysis with balloon angioplasty in the 1980s, the combined recanalization strategy with modern PCI was not compromised by early reocclusion or bleeding (72–77).

The need to revisit the question of management of STEMI in terms other than either primary PCI or thrombolysis is underscored not only by results from these trials. Even if one accepts the superiority of primary PCI to thrombolysis when it can be performed in a timely fashion (49,71), the issue of time to reperfusion is not obviated. Single centers have found mechanisms to effectively reduce door-to-balloon times for primary PCI (78). Yet nationally it has been possible to reduce door-to-balloon times by only 8 minutes during the entire past decade (59,60). The central importance of rapid induction of reperfusion for patients with STEMI is reemphasized by recent findings from the PAMI trials (Fig. 1.5) (36,79). A greater than fivefold increase in late mortality was seen in patients in whom therapy before PCI did not induce TIMI grade 3 flow at the time of initial angiography (79). Insights from PACT and PAMI are thus congruent with respect to the importance of prompt, early reperfusion (even in patients subsequently being managed invasively); so are several other trials that demonstrated remarkably low mortality in patients treated with thrombolytic drugs very early after onset of STEMI (80–82).

In aggregate, available results suggest an important role for early, pharmacologically induced reperfusion regardless of subsequent measures including PCI. They lead to consideration of a "new" question: What is the best pharmacological approach to establish complete, early reperfusion that can be combined with subsequent PCI to broaden the temporal window during which recanalization can safely maximize

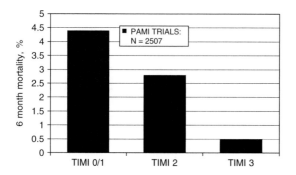

Figure 1.5 Improved survival in patients undergoing primary PCI is dependent not only on final TIMI grade 3 flow. The presence or absence of patency of the artery early, i.e., at the time of presentation in the catheterization laboratory, presages low or high mortality for patients undergoing primary PCI. (From Ref. 79.)

early and long-term outcomes? Asking this question brings us "back to the future," i.e., full circle to the 1980s and to the initial marriage of invasive and thrombolytic approaches (Fig. 1.6). Rather than asking whether the cardiac catheterization laboratory is needed to deliver thrombolytic agents (13), we must ask whether the interventionalist can now provide the means to definitively "rescue" (72–77) and/or sustain culprit artery patency when thrombolysis has yielded suboptimal TIMI grade flow or been accompanied by significant residual stenosis. Although it is possible that glycoprotein (GP) IIb/IIIa inhibitors alone may constitute conjunctive therapy for PCI in the treatment of STEMI (83), these agents have limited efficacy in establishing TIMI grade 3 flow before implementation of PCI (84). Furthermore, a mortality benefit for GP IIb/IIIa inhibitors in the treatment of STEMI has not been established (56,85). Fibrinolysis (with or without conjunctive GP IIb/IIIa inhibition) is the best current pharmacological option for inducing TIMI grade 3 flow. It seems likely that the combination of fibrinolysis followed by early PCI to completely and definitively recanalize the infarct-related artery constitutes an attractive option. The option is especially attractive for the many patients with STEMI for whom a

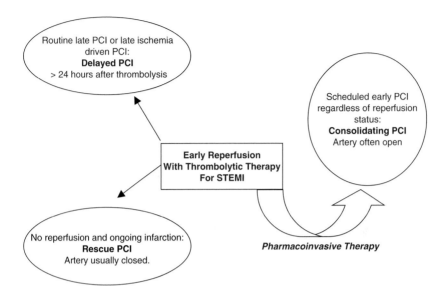

Figure 1.6   Can reperfusion be established before PCI can be implemented for patients with STEMI? Although a rescue PCI strategy is one commonly used, as is a late (>24 hours post-AMI) PCI strategy, pharmacoinvasive therapy with consolidating PCI may combine the best features of induction of reperfusion early with sustained and complete reperfusion achievable with the two techniques applied in tandem for the large majority of patients with STEMI.

90-minute interval from the hospitalization to open artery by primary PCI is impossible because of limitations of transport (30, 86, 87).

VIII.   THE OPTIMAL PHARMACOINVASIVE APPROACH

Three types of pharmacoinvasive therapy are being utilized currently:

    1.   Thrombolysis followed as promptly as possible by PCI for all patients with STEMI who do not have an absolute contraindication to fibrinolysis. This modality has been referred to by others as "facilitated PCI" (73) although, as noted above, thrombolysis does not, in fact, facilitate PCI. Because PCI

early after thrombolysis can establish recanalization when
lysis has failed and can consolidate benefit when it has suc-
ceeded, we prefer to refer to it as consolidating PCI.

2.   Thrombolysis followed by PCI in patients in whom throm-
     bolysis has failed, referred to as rescue PCI (72).

3.   Thrombolysis followed by late PCI, if needed, to ameliorate
     recurrent ischemia before discharge from the hospital,
     referred to as delayed PCI (88).

Nearly 80% of patients with STEMI in the United States undergo
cardiac catheterization during an index hospitalization (88). In the
worldwide GRACE registry, results with this approach appeared to be
favorable (89) and consistent with the recent results of studies such as
SPEED and PACT (73,74). The optimal combination and timing of the
pharmacologic and technologic arms of pharmacoinvasive therapy
remain to be determined. Trials such as ASSENT III and GUSTO V
have shown that the benefits (reduced incidence of reinfarction with
enoxaparin or GP IIb/IIIa inhibitors) and limitations (increased bleeding in elderly patients when GP IIb/IIIa inhibitors and enoxaparin are
used concomitantly with fibrinolytic agents) encountered with specific
conjunctive regimens may limit the extent to which pharmacological
regimens alone can further improve outcomes (65,66,90). However,
anticoagulants and antiplatelet agents under development with novel
modes of action may overcome these limitations. Results of trials in
progress (i.e., ASSENT IV and FINESSE) should help to define the
timing of PCI after thrombolysis that will improve survival of patients
with STEMI hospitalized at sites with or without capabilities for coronary angiography (91).

Optimal pharmacoinvasive therapy should achieve the following:
(a) prompt induction of reperfusion (within the "golden" 2 hours after
onset of chest pain indicative of ischemia); (b) subsequent induction
of complete reperfusion; (c) sustained reperfusion; and (d) avoidance
of reinfarction or bleeding. The specific regimens and timing for use
of the two components entailed will require further study in randomized
clinical trials. Recommendations can be made even now, however, in
light of well-established principles and outcomes.

- Initial fibrinolytic therapy (in patients who have no absolute contraindication to thrombolysis) should be combined with administration of conjunctive pharmacological agents to enhance lysis and minimize the risk of bleeding.
- Appropriate pharmacological regimens include full- or half-dose fibrinolytic drugs with enoxaparin (65,92) or GP IIb/IIIa inhibitors (65,66,68). The high rate of bleeding with conjunctive GP IIb/IIIa inhibitors, especially in elderly patients, may favor use of a full dose of the fibrinolytic agent with unfractionated heparin (65), particularly in view of adverse events in elderly patients treated with full-dose tenectophase and enoxaparin (90). Optimal regimens for pharmacological treatment of elderly patients with STEMI remain to be defined (93).

The benefits of conjunctive GP IIb/IIIa inhibitors and enoxaparin in GUSTO V and ASSENT 3 were confined to reduction of the incidence of reinfarction. Because reinfarction occurs on an average of 2.2 days following STEMI (94), it is not clear that an increased bleeding risk entailed with the use of these agents is acceptable if PCI can be used to reduce the risk of reinfarction on a regular basis (77). Whether any increased risk of bleeding is tolerable or necessary will likely depend upon the availability of early PCI (Fig. 1.7).

- If a patient has a contraindication to fibrinolysis, transfer for urgent PCI should occur immediately (95). Even in this setting, pharmacological therapy with a GP IIb/IIIa inhibitor can be initiated before PCI. Pharmacological therapy can exert a favorable impact on early outcome by facilitating establishment of early, though limited, patency of the infarct-related artery in patients subsequently undergoing acute infarct PCI (84,96).
- Aggressive use of rescue PCI for patients with incomplete, early recanalization reduces mortality (72,76). Thus, after prompt initiation of pharmacological therapy, early PCI should be considered for all patients with STEMI who meet criteria for potentially beneficial rescue PCI, including the presence of ongoing symptoms or ST segment elevation persisting

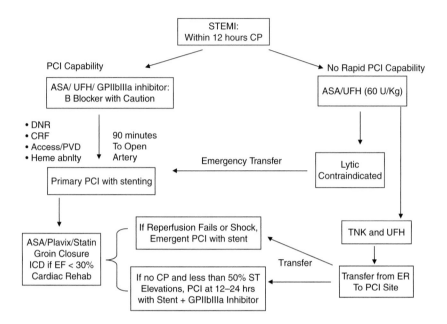

Figure 1.7   A sample algorithm for invasive and noninvasive hospitals caring for patients with STEMI and utilizing primary, rescue, and pharmacoinvasive approaches.

for 60 minutes or more after the onset of pharmacological coronary thrombolysis.

- Pharmacoinvasive recanalization with fibrinolytic therapy to induce initial reperfusion, conjunctive pharmacological therapy with anticoagulants to enhance the rapidity and extent of lysis and subsequent timely (within 12–24 hours) PCI to prevent reocclusion and reinfarction to eliminate underlying anatomical obstruction and thrombus are particularly promising for most patients with STEMI (30,73–77). This pharmacoinvasive approach for treatment of asymptomatic patients following thrombolysis should expand the interval during which PCI can be effective well beyond the 90-minute interval within which optimal benefits are seen with primary PCI. If so, it would be attractive for patients presenting to

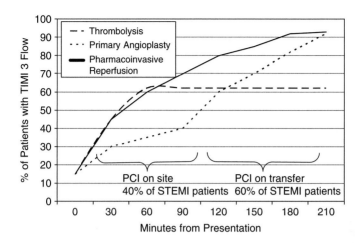

Figure 1.8 A hypothetical cumulative frequency distribution of time to Thrombolysis In Myocardial Infarction (TIMI) grade 3 flow in patients treated for ST segment elevation myocardial infarction. Although as many as 50% of patients can be expected to exhibit TIMI 3 flow induced with thrombolysis in the first 60 minutes after hospital presentation, achievement of TIMI grade 3 flow in 90% of patients with STEMI requires a pharmacoinvasive recanalization strategy and a broadening of the window during which benefit can be conferred. (From Ref. 30.)

tertiary care facilities and certainly also for those requiring transfer to such facilities (Fig. 1.7).

We believe that pharmacoinvasive therapy has the potential to combine the best aspects of both pharmacologically and interventionally induced and sustained reperfusion (Fig. 1.8). Its potential should, of course, be the focus of debate and hence investigation. Contrasting the merits of thrombolysis with those of primary PCI should not.

REFERENCES

1. Maroko PR, Kjekshus JK, Sobel BE, Watanabe T, Covell JW, Ross J Jr, Braunwald E. Factors influencing infarct size following experimental coronary artery occlusions. Circulation 1971; 43:67–82.

2. Sobel BE, Bresnahan GF, Shell WE, Yoder RD. Estimation of infarct size in man and its relation to prognosis. Circulation 1972; 46:640–648.

3. Swan HJ, Forrester JS, Diamond G, Chatterjee K, Parmley WW. Hemodynamic spectrum of myocardial infarction and cardiogenic shock. A conceptual model. Circulation 1972; 45:1097–1110.

4. Forrester JS, Chatterjee K, Jobin G. A new conceptual approach to the therapy of acute myocardial infarction. Adv Cardiol 1975; 15:111–123.

5. Shell WE, Sobel BE. Protection of jeopardized ischemic myocardium by reduction of ventricular afterload. N Engl J Med 1974; 291:481– 486.

6. Maroko PR, Libby P, Ginks WR, Bloor CM, Shell WE, Sobel BE, Ross J Jr. Coronary artery reperfusion. I. Early effects on local myocardial function and the extent of myocardial necrosis. J Clin Invest 1972; 51:2710–2716.

7. Fletcher AP, Alkjaersig N, Smyrniotis FE, Sherry S. The treatment of patients suffering from early myocardial infarction with massive and prolonged streptokinase therapy. Trans Assoc Am Phys 1958; 71:287–296.

8. Bett JH, Castaldi PA, Hale GS, Isbister JP, McLean KH, O'Sullivan EF, Biggs JC, Chesterman CN, Hirsh J, McDonald IG, Morgan JJ, Rosenbaum M. Australian multicentre trial of streptokinase in acute myocardial infarction. Lancet 1973; 1:57–60.

9. European Working Party. Streptokinase in recent myocardial infarction: a controlled multicentre trial. Br Med J 1971; 3:325–331.

10. Stampfer MJ, Goldhaber SZ, Yusuf S, Peto R, Hennekens CH. Effect of intravenous streptokinase on acute myocardial infarction: pooled results from randomized trials. N Engl J Med 1982; 307:1180–1182.

11. European Cooperative Study Group for Streptokinase Treatment in Acute Myocardial Infarction. Streptokinase in acute myocardial infarction. N Engl J Med 1979; 301:797–802.

12. Chazov EI, Matveeva LS, Mazaev AV, Sargin KE, Sadovskaia GV, Ruda MI. Intracoronary administration of fibrinolysin in acute myocardial infarct. Ter Arkh 1976; 48:8–19.

13. Rentrop KP, Blanke H, Karsch KR, Wiegand V, Kostering H, Oster H, Leitz K. Acute myocardial infarction: intracoronary application of nitroglycerin and streptokinase. Clin Cardiol 1979; 2:354–363.

14. Bergmann SR, Lerch RA, Fox KAA, Ludbrook PA, Welch MJ, Ter-Pogossian MM, Sobel BE. Temporal dependence of beneficial effects of coronary thrombolysis characterized by positron tomography. Am J Med 1982; 73:573–581.

15. Collen D, Topol EJ, Tiefenbrunn AJ, Gold HK, Weisfeldt ML, Sobel BE, Leinbach RC, Brinker JA, Ludbrook PA, Yasuda I, Bulkley BH, Robison AK, Hutter AM Jr, Bell WR, Spadaro JJ Jr, Khaw BA, Grossbard EB. Coronary thrombolysis with recombinant human tissue-type plasminogen activator: a prospective, randomized, placebo-controlled trial. Circulation 1984; 70:1012–1017.

16. TIMI Study Group. The Thrombolysis in Myocardial Infarction (TIMI) trial. Phase I findings. N Engl J Med 1985; 312:932–936.

17. Verstraete M, Bernard R, Bory M, Brower RW, Collen D, deBono DP, Erbel R, Huhmann W, Lennane RJ, Lubsen J, et al. Randomised trial of intravenous recombinant tissue-type plasminogen activator versus intravenous streptokinase in acute myocardial infarction. Report from the European Cooperative Study Group for Recombinant Tissue-type Plasminogen Activator. Lancet 1985; 1:842–847.

18. Van de Werf F, Ludbrook PA, Bergmann SR, Tiefenbrunn AJ, Fox KAA, de Geest H, Verstraete M, Collen D, Sobel BE. Coronary thrombolysis with tissue-type plasminogen activator in patients with evolving myocardial infarction. N Engl J Med 1984; 310:609–613.

19. Gruppo Italiano per lo Studio della Streptochinasi nell'Infarto Miocardico (GISSI). Effectiveness of intravenous thrombolytic treatment in acute myocardial infarction. Lancet 1986; 1:397–402.

20. AIMS Trial Study Group. Effect of intravenous APSAC on mortality after acute myocardial infarction: preliminary report of a placebo-controlled clinical trial. Lancet 1988; 1:545–549.

21. ISIS-2. ISIS-2 (Second International Study of Infarct Survival) Collaborative Group. Randomised trial of intravenous streptokinase, oral aspirin, both, or neither among 17,187 cases of suspected acute myocardial infarction: Lancet 1988; 2:349–360.

22. Wilcox RG, von der Lippe G, Olsson CG, Jensen G, Skene AM, Hampton JR. Trial of tissue plasminogen activator for mortality reduction in acute myocardial infarction. Anglo-Scandinavian Study of Early Thrombolysis (ASSET). Lancet 1988; 2:525–530.

23. National Heart Foundation of Australia Coronary Thrombolysis Group. Coronary thrombolysis and myocardial salvage by tissue plasminogen activator given up to 4 hours after onset of myocardial infarction. Lancet 1988; 1:203–208.

24. Kennedy JW, Ritchie JL, Davis KB, Fritz JK. Western Washington randomized trial of intracoronary streptokinase in acute myocardial infarction. N Engl J Med 1983; 309:1477–1482.

25. Sobel BE. Angioplasty or thrombolysis: misconstrued questions and misleading answers. Coron Artery Dis 1996; 7:933–934.

26. Topol EJ, Califf RM, George BS, Kereiakes DJ, Abbottsmith CW, Candela RJ, Lee KL, Pitt B, Stack RS, O'Neill WW. A randomized trial of immediate versus delayed elective angioplasty after intravenous tissue plasminogen activator in acute myocardial infarction. N Engl J Med 1987; 317:581–588.

27. The TIMI Study Group. Comparison of invasive and conservative strategies after treatment with intravenous tissue plasminogen activator in acute myocardial infarction. Results of the thrombolysis in myocardial infarction (TIMI) phase II trial. N Engl J Med 1989; 320:618–627.

28. Simoons ML, Arnold AE, Betriu A, de Bono DP, Col J, Dougherty FC, von Essen R, Lambertz H, Lubsen J, Meier B, et al. Thrombolysis with tissue plasminogen activator in acute myocardial infarction: no additional benefit from immediate percutaneous coronary angioplasty. Lancet 1988; 1:197–203.

29. Passamani E, Hodges M, Herman M, Grose R, Chaitman B, Rogers W, Forman S, Terrin M, Knatterud G, Robertson T, et al. The Thrombolysis in Myocardial Infarction (TIMI) phase II pilot study: tissue plasminogen activator followed by percutaneous transluminal coronary angioplasty. J Am Coll Cardiol 1987; 10:51B–64B.

30. Dauerman HL, Sobel BE. Synergistic treatment of ST-segment elevation myocardial infarction with pharmacoinvasive recanalization. J Am Coll Cardiol 2003; 42:646–651.

31. Weaver WD, Cerqueira M, Hallstrom AP, Litwin PE, Martin JS, Kudenchuk PJ, Eisenberg M. Prehospital-initiated vs. hospital-initiated thrombolytic thereapy. The Myocardial Infarction Triage and Intervention Trial. JAMA 1993; 270:1211–1216.

32. Tiefenbrunn AJ, Sobel BE. Timing of coronary recanalization. Paradigms, paradoxes, and pertinence. Circulation 1992; 85:2311–2315.

33. Zijlstra F, Patel A, Jones M, Grines CL, Ellis S, Garcia E, Grinfeld L, Gibbons RJ, Ribeiro EE, Ribichini F, Granger C, Akhras F, Weaver WD, Simes RJ. Clinical characteristics and outcome of patients with early (<2 h), intermediate (2–4 h) and late (>4 h) presentation treated by primary coronary angioplasty or thrombolytic therapy for acute myocardial infarction. Eur Heart J 2002; 23:550–557.

34. Berger PB, Ellis SG, Holmes DR, Jr, Granger CB, Criger DA, Betriu A, Topol EJ, Califf RM. Relationship between delay in performing direct coronary angioplasty and early clinical outcome in patients with acute myocardial infarction: results from the global use of strategies to open occluded arteries in Acute Coronary Syndromes (GUSTO-IIb) trial. Circulation 1999; 100:14–20.

35. Brodie BR, Kissling G. Relationship between delay in performing direct coronary angioplasty and early clinical outcome in patients with acute myocardial infarction. Circulation 2000; 102:E29–E30.

36. Brodie BR, Stone GW, Morice MC, Cox DA, Garcia E, Mattos LA, Boura J, O'Neill WW, Stuckey TD, Milks S, Lansky AJ, Grines CL. Stent Primary Angioplasty in Myocardial Infarction Study Group. Importance of time to reperfusion on outcomes with primary coronary angioplasty for acute myocardial infarction (results from the Stent Primary Angioplasty in Myocardial Infarction Trial). Am J Cardiol 2001; 88:1085–1090.

37. Furman MI, Dauerman HL, Goldberg RJ, Yarzebski J, Lessard D, Gore JM. Twenty-two year (1975 to 1997) trends in the incidence, in-hospital and long-term case fatality rates from initial Q-wave and non-Q-wave myocardial infarction: a multi-hospital, community-wide perspective. J Am Coll Cardiol 2001; 37:1571–1580.

38. Dauerman HL, Lessard D, Yarzebski J, Furman MI, Gore JM, Goldberg RJ. Ten-year trends in the incidence, treatment, and outcome of Q-wave myocardial infarction. Am J Cardiol 2000; 86:730–735.

39. The GUSTO Angiographic Investigators. The effects of tissue plasminogen activator, streptokinase, or both on coronary-artery patency, ventricular function, and survival after acute myocardial infarction. N Engl J Med 1993; 329:1615–1622.

40. Lenderink T, Simoons ML, Van Es GA, Van de Werf F, Verstraete M, Arnold AE. Benefit of thrombolytic therapy is sustained throughout five years and is related to TIMI perfusion grade 3 but not grade 2 flow at discharge. The European Cooperative Study Group. Circulation 1995; 92:1110–1116.

41. The Global Use of Strategies to Open Occluded Coronary Arteries in Acute Coronary Syndromes (GUSTO IIb) Angioplasty Substudy Investigators. A clinical trial comparing primary coronary angioplasty with tissue plasminogen activator for acute myocardial infarction. N Engl J Med 1997; 336:1621–1628.

42. Anderson JL, Karagounis LA, Becker LC, Sorensen SG, Menlove RL. TIMI perfusion grade 3 but not grade 2 results in improved outcome after thrombolysis for myocardial infarction. Ventriculographic, enzymatic, and electrocardiographic evidence from the TEAM-3 Study. Circulation 1993; 87:1829–1839.

43. Meyer J, Merx W, Schmitz H, Erbel R, Kiesslich T, Dorr R, Lambertz H, Bethge C, Krebs W, Bardos P, Minale C, Messmer BJ, Effert S. Percutaneous transluminal coronary angioplasty immediately after intracoronary streptolysis of transmural myocardial infarction. Circulation 1982; 66:905–913.

44. O'Neill W, Timmis GC, Bourdillon PD, Lai P, Ganghadarhan V, Walton J Jr, Ramos R, Laufer N, Gordon S, Schork MA, et al. A prospective randomized clinical trial of intracoronary streptokinase versus coronary angioplasty for acute myocardial infarction. N Engl J Med 1986; 314: 812–818.

45. Zijlstra F, de Boer MJ, Hoorntje JC, Reiffers S, Reiber JH, Suryapranata H. A comparison of immediate coronary angioplasty with intravenous streptokinase in acute myocardial infarction. N Engl J Med 1993; 328:680–684.

46. Grines CL, Browne KF, Marco J, Rothbaum D, Stone GW, O'Keefe J, Overlie P, Donohue B, Chelliah N, Timmis GC, et al. A comparison of immediate angioplasty with thrombolytic therapy for acute myocardial infarction. The Primary Angioplasty in Myocardial Infarction Study Group. N Engl J Med 1993; 328:673–679.

47. Ryan TJ, Ryan TJ, Jr., Jacobs AK. Primary PTCA versus thrombolytic therapy: an evidence-based summary. Am Heart J 1999; 138:S96–104.

48. Ryan TJ, Antman EM, Brooks NH, Califf RM, Hillis LD, Hiratzka LF, Rapaport E, Riegel B, Russell RO, Smith EE III, Weaver WD, Gibbons RJ, Alpert JS, Eagle KA, Gardner TJ, Garson A Jr, Gregoratos G, Ryan TG, Smith SC Jr. 1999 update: ACC/AHA guidelines for the management of patients with acute myocardial infarction. A report of the American College of Cardiology/American Heart Association Task Force on Practice Guidelines (Committee on Management of Acute Myocardial Infarction). J Am Coll Cardiol 1999; 34:890–911.

49. Weaver WD, Simes RJ, Betriu A, Grines CL, Zijlstra F, Garcia E, Grinfeld L, Gibbons RJ, Ribeiro EE, DeWood MA, Ribichini F. Comparison of primary coronary angioplasty and intravenous thrombolytic therapy for acute myocardial infarction: a quantitative review. JAMA 1997; 278:2093–2098.

50. Tiefenbrunn AJ, Chandra NC, French WJ, Gore JM, Rogers WJ. Clinical experience with primary percutaneous transluminal coronary angioplasty compared with alteplase (recombinant tissue-type plasminogen activator) in patients with acute myocardial infarction: a report from the Second National Registry of Myocardial Infarction (NRMI-2). J Am Coll Cardiol 1998; 31:1240–1245.

51. Danchin N, Vaur L, Genes N, Etienne S, Angioi M, Ferrieres J, Cambou JP. Treatment of acute myocardial infarction by primary coronary angioplasty or intravenous thrombolysis in the "real world": one-year results from a nationwide French survey. Circulation 1999; 99:2639–2644.

52. Dauerman HL, Pinto DS, Ho KK, Gibson CM, Kuntz RE, Cohen DJ, Baim DS, Carrozza JP Jr. Outcome of patients with acute myocardial infarction who are ineligible for primary angioplasty trials. Catheter Cardiovasc Interv 2000; 49:237–243.

53. Cannon CP, Gibson CM, Lambrew CT, Shoultz DA, Levy D, French WJ, Gore JM, Weaver WD, Rogers WJ, Tiefenbrunn AJ. Relationship of symptom-onset-to-balloon time and door-to-balloon time with mortality in patients undergoing angioplasty for acute myocardial infarction. JAMA 2000; 283:2941–2947.

54. Canto JG, Every NR, Magid DJ, Rogers WJ, Malmgren JA, Frederick PD, French WJ, Tiefenbrunn AJ, Misra VK, Kiefe CI, Barron HV. The volume of primary angioplasty procedures and survival after acute

myocardial infarction. National Registry of Myocardial Infarction 2 Investigators. N Engl J Med 2000; 342:1573–1580.

55. Magid DJ, Calonge BN, Rumsfeld JS, Canto JG, Frederick PD, Every NR, Barron HV: National Registry of Myocardial Infarction 2 and 3 Investigators. Relation between hospital primary angioplasty volume and mortality for patients with acute MI treated with primary angioplasty vs. thrombolytic therapy. JAMA 2000; 284:3131–3138.

56. Stone GW, Grines CL, Cox DA, Garcia E, Txheng JE, Griffin JJ, Guagliumi G, Stuckey T, Turco M, Carrool JD, Rutherford BD, Lansky AJ: Controlled Abciximab and Device Investigation to Lower Late Angioplasty Complications (CADILLAC) Investigators. Comparison of angioplasty with stenting, with or without abciximab, in acute myocardial infarction. N Engl J Med 2002; 346:957–966.

57. Aversano T, Aversano LT, Passamani E, Knatterud GL, Terrin ML, Williams DO, Forman SA: Atlantic Cardiovascular Patient Outcomes Research Team (C-PORT). Thrombolytic therapy vs. primary percutaneous coronary intervention for myocardial infarction in patients presenting to hospitals without on-site cardiac surgery: a randomized controlled trial. JAMA 2002; 287:1943–1951.

58. Anderson HR. The DANAMI-2 Study. Paper presented at Late Breaking Clinical Trials Sessions of the American College of Cardiology, Atlanta, GA, March 20, 2002.

59. Angeja BG, Gibson CM, Chin R, Frederick PD, Every NR, Ross AM, Stone GW, Barron HV: Participants in the National Registry of Myocardial Infarction 2-3. Predictors of door-to-balloon delay in primary angioplasty. Am J Cardiol 2002; 89:1156–1161.

60. Gibson CM. Time is myocardium and time is outcomes. Circulation 2001; 104:2632–2634.

61. Angeja BG, Gunda M, Murphy SA, Sobe BE Rundle AC, Syed M, Asfour A, Borzak S, Gourlay SG, Barron HV, Gibbons RJ, Gibson CM. TIMI myocardial perfusion grade and ST segment resolution: association with infarct size as assessed by single photon emission computed tomography imaging. Circulation 2002; 105:282–285.

62. An international randomized trial comparing four thrombolytic strategies for acute myocardial infarction. The GUSTO investigators. N Engl J Med 1993; 329:673–682.

63. Fox KAA, Robison AK, Knabb RM, Rosamond TL, Sobel BE, Bergmann SR. Prevention of coronary thrombosis with subthrombolytic doses of tissue-type plasminogen activator. Circulation 1985; 72:1346– 1354.

64. Barbash GI, Birnbaum Y, Bogaerts K, Hudson M, Lesaffre E, Fu Y, Goodman S, Houbracken K, Munsters K, Granger CB, Pieper K, Califf RM, Topol EJ, Van De Werf F. Treatment of reinfarction after thrombolytic therapy for acute myocardial infarction: an analysis of outcome and treatment choices in the global utilization of streptokinase and tissue plasminogen activator for occluded coronary arteries (gusto I) and assessment of the safety of a new thrombolytic (assent 2) studies. Circulation 2001; 103:954–960.

65. Efficacy and safety of tenecteplase in combination with enoxaparin, abciximab, or unfractionated heparin: the ASSENT-3 randomised trial in acute myocardial infarction. Lancet 2001; 358:605–613.

66. Topol EJ. Reperfusion therapy for acute myocardial infarction with fibrinolytic therapy or combination reduced fibrinolytic therapy and platelet glycoprotein IIb/IIIa inhibition: the GUSTO V randomised trial. Lancet 2001; 357:1905–1914.

67. Sobel BE, Hirsh J. Principles and practice of coronary thrombolysis and conjunctive treatment. Am J Cardiol 1991; 68:382–388.

68. Ohman EM, Kleiman NS, Gacioch G, Worley SJ, Navetta FI, Talley JD, Anderson HV, Ellis SG, Cohen MD, Spriggs D, Miller M, Kereiakes D, Yakubov S, Kitt MM, Sigmon KN, Califf RM, Krucoff MW, Topol EJ. Combined accelerated tissue-plasminogen activator and platelet glycoprotein IIb/IIIa integrin receptor blockade with Integrilin in acute myocardial infarction. Results of a randomized, placebo-controlled, dose-ranging trial. IMPACT-AMI Investigators. Circulation 1997; 95:846–854.

69. Grines CL, Westerhausen DR, Jr., Grines LL, Hanlon JT, Logemann TL, Niemela M, Weaver WD, Graham M, Boura J, O'Neill WW, Balestrini C: Air PAMI Study Group. A randomized trial of transfer for primary angioplasty versus on-site thrombolysis in patients with high-risk myocardial infarction: the Air Primary Angioplasty in Myocardial Infarction study. J Am Coll Cardiol 2002; 39:1713–1719.

70. Schomig A, Ndrepepa G, Mehilli J, Schwaiger M, Schuhlen H, Nekolla S, Pache J, Martinoff S, Bollwein H, Kastrati A. Therapy-dependent

influence of time-to-treatment interval on myocardial salvage in patients with acute myocardial infarction treated with coronary artery stenting or thrombolysis. Circulation 2003; 108:1084–1088.

71. Van de Werf F, Baim DS. Reperfusion for ST-segment elevation myocardial infarction: an overview of current treatment options. Circulation 2002; 105:2813–2816.

72. Schomig A, Ndrepepa G, Mehilli J, Dirschinger J, Nekoll SG, Schmitt C, Martinoff S, Seyfarth M, Schwaiger M, Kastrati A. A randomized trial of coronary stenting versus balloon angioplasty as a rescue intervention after failed thrombolysis in patients with acute myocardial infarction. J Am Coll Cardiol 2004; 44:2073–2079.

73. Herrmann HC, Moliterno DJ, Ohman EM, Stebbins AL, Bode C, Betriu A, Forycki F, Miklin JS, Bachinsky WB, Lincoff AM, Califf RM, Topol EJ. Facilitation of early percutaneous coronary intervention after reteplase with or without abciximab in acute myocardial infarction: results from the SPEED (GUSTO-4 Pilot) Trial. J Am Coll Cardiol 2000; 36:1489–1496.

74. Ross AM, Coyne KS, Reiner JS, Greenhouse SW, Fink C, Frey A, Moreyra E, Traboulsi M, Racine N, Riba AL, Thompson MA, Rohrbeck S, Lundergan CF. A randomized trial comparing primary angioplasty with a strategy of short-acting thrombolysis and immediate planned rescue angioplasty in acute myocardial infarction: the PACT trial. PACT investigators. Plasminogen-activator Angioplasty Compatibility Trial. J Am Coll Cardiol 1999; 34:1954–1962.

75. Dauerman HL, Prpic R, Andreou C, Popma JJ. Resolution of coronary thrombus with rescue stenting. Am J Cardiol 2000; 85:1244–1247.

76. Schweiger MJ, Cannon CP, Murphy SA, Gibson CM, Cook JR, Giugliano RP, Changezi HU, Antman EM, Braunwald E: TIMI 10B and TIMI 14 Investigators. Early coronary intervention following pharmacological therapy for acute myocardial infarction (the combined TIMI 10B-TIMI 14 experience). Am J Cardiol 2001; 88:831–836.

77. Scheller B, Hennen B, Hammer B, Walle J, Hofer C, Hilpert V, Winter I, Nickenig G, Bohm M, SIAM III Study Group. Beneficial effects of immediate stenting after thrombolysis in acute myocardial infarction. J Am Coll Cardiol 2003; 42:634–641.

78. Caputo RP, Ho KK, Stoler RC, Sukin CA, Lopez JJ, Cohen DJ, Kuntz RE, Berman A, Carrozza JP, Baim DS. Effect of continuous quality improvement analysis on the delivery of primary percutaneous transluminal coronary angioplasty for acute myocardial infarction. Am J Cardiol 1997; 79:1159–1164.

79. Stone GW, Cox D, Garcia E, Brodie BR, Morice MC, Griffin J, Mattos L, Lansky AJ, O'Neill WW, Grines CL. Normal flow (TIMI 3) before mechanical reperfusion therapy is an independent determinant of survival in acute myocardial infarction: analysis from the primary angioplasty in myocardial infarction trials. Circulation 2001; 104:636–641.

80. Rozenman Y, Gotsman MS, Weiss AT, Lotan C, Mosseri M, Sapoznikov D, Welber S, Hasin Y, Gilon D. Early intravenous thrombolysis in acute myocardial infaraction: the Jerusalem experience. Int J Cardiol 1995; 49:S21–S28.

81. Binbrek A, Rao N, Absher PM, Van de Werf F, Sobel BE. The relative rapidity of recanalization induced by recombinant tissue-type plasminogen activator (rt-PA) and TNK-tPA assessed with enzymatic methods. Coron Artery Dis 2000; 11:429–435.

82. Bonnefoy E, Lapostolle F, Leizorovicz A, Steg G, McFadden EP, Dubien PY, Cattan S, Boullenger E, Machecourt J, Lacroute J-M, Cassagnes J, Dissait F, Touboul P for The Comparison of Angioplasty and Prehospital Thrombolysis in Acute Myocardial Infarction (CAPTIM) Study Group. Primary angioplasty versus prehospital fibrinolysis in acute myocardial infarction: a randomized study. Lancet 2002; 360: 825–829.

83. Brener SJ, Barr LA, Burchenal JE, Katz S, George BS, Jones AA, Cohen ED, Gainey PC, White HJ, Cheek HB, Moses JW, Moliterno DJ, Effron MB, Topol EJ. Randomized, placebo-controlled trial of platelet glycoprotein IIb/IIIa blockade with primary angioplasty for acute myocardial infarction. ReoPro and Primary PTCA Organization and Randomized Trial (RAPPORT) Investigators. Circulation 1998; 98:734–741.

84. Cutlip DE, Cove CJ, Irons D, Kalaria V, Le M, Cronmiller H, Caufield L, Pomerantz RM, Ling FS. Emergency room administration of eptifibatide before primary angioplasty for ST elevation acute myocardial infarction and its effect on baseline coronary flow and procedure outcomes. Am J Cardiol 2001; 88:A6, 62–64.

85. Eisenberg MJ, Jamal S. Glycoprotein IIb/IIIa inhibition in the setting of acute ST-segment elevation myocardial infarction. J Am Coll Cardiol 2003; 42:1–6.

86. Sobel BE. Interpretation of results of clinical trials in coronary thrombolysis. Fibrinolysis Proteolysis 1997; 11:17–21.

87. Dauerman HL. The early days after ST-segment elevation acute myocardial infarction: reconsidering the delayed invasive approach. J Am Coll Cardiol 2003; 42:420–423.

88. Spencer FA, Goldberg RJ, Frederick PD, Malmgren J, Becker RC, Gore JM. Age and the utilization of cardiac catheterization following uncomplicated first acute myocardial infarction treated with thrombolytic therapy (The Second National Registry of Myocardial Infarction [NRMI-2]). Am J Cardiol 2001; 88:107–111.

89. Saddiq I, Dauerman HL, Goldberg RJ, Klein W, Brieger D, Steg PG, Montalescot G, Lopez-Sendon J, Budaj A, Gore J. Post thrombolytic management of acute myocardial infarction: Insights from the Global Registry of Acute Coronary Events (GRACE). Am J Cardiol 2002; 90:190H.

90. Wallentin L, Goldstein P, Armstrong PW, Granger CB, Adgey AA, Arntz HR, Bogaerts K, Danays T, Lindahl B, Makijarvi M, Vergeugt F, Van de Werf F. Efficacy and safety of tenecteplase in combination with the low-molecular-weight heparin enoxaparin or unfractionated heparin in the prehospital setting: the Assessment of the Safety and Efficacy of a New Thrombolytic Regimen (ASSENT)-3PLUS randomized trial in acute myocardial infarction. Circulation 203; 108:135–142.

91. Mehta RH, Criger DA, Granger CB, Pieper KK, Califf RM, Topol EJ, Bates ER. Patient outcomes after fibrinolytic therapy for acute myocardial infarction at hospitals with and without coronary revascularization capability. J Am Coll Cardiol 2002; 40:1034–1040.

92. Antman EM, Louwerenburg HW, Baars HF, Wesdorp JC, Hamer B, Bassand JP, Bigonzi F, Pisapia G, Gibson CM, Heidbuchel H, Braunwald E, Van de Werf F. Enoxaparin as adjunctive antithrombin therapy for ST-elevation myocardial infarction: results of the ENTIRE-Thrombolysis in Myocardial Infarction (TIMI) 23 Trial. Circulation 2002; 105:1642–1649.

93. White HD. Thrombolytic therapy in the elderly. Lancet 2001; 357: 1367–1368.

94. Gibson CM, Karha J, Murphy SA, James D, Morrow DA, Cannon CP, Giugliano RP, Antman EM, Braunwald E, for the TIMI Study Group. Early and long-term clinical outcomes associated with reinfarction following fibrinolytic administration in the Thrombolysis in Myocardial Infarction trials. J Am Coll Cardiol 2003; 42:7–16.

95. Hochman JS, Buller CE, Sleeper LA, Boland J, Dzavik V, Sanborn TA, Godfrey E, White HD, Lim J, LeJemtel T. Cardiogenic shock complicating acute myocardial infarction-etiologies, management and outcome: a report from the SHOCK Trial Registry. Should we emergently revascularize occluded coronaries for cardiogenic shock? J Am Coll Cardiol 2000; 36:1063–1070.

96. Antoniucci D, Valenti R, Migliorini A, Moschi G, Trapani M, Dovellini EV, Bolognese L, Santoro GM. Abciximab therapy improves survival in patients with acute myocardial infarction complicated by early cardiogenic shock undergoing coronary artery stent implantation. Am J Cardiol 2002; 90:353–357.

2

Development, Impact, and Limitations of Coronary Thrombolysis: Milestones in Pharmacological Reperfusion Therapy

ALAN J. TIEFENBRUNN

Washington University in St. Louis
St. Louis, Missouri, U.S.A.

I. INTRODUCTION

Many factors have contributed to the decline in cardiovascular-related mortality over the past quarter century, including lifestyle modifications, the development of multiple new drug categories, the introduction and subsequent dramatic improvements in percutaneous coronary intervention (PCI), cardiac transplantation, and advances in electrophysiology and implantable devices. One of the more important new treatments is reperfusion therapy for patients with evolving acute myocardial infarction (AMI), which has now become the standard of care for these individuals. This chapter will review selected major developments in historical perspective that led to the widespread application of pharmacological reperfusion therapy for the treatment of AMI (Fig. 2.1).

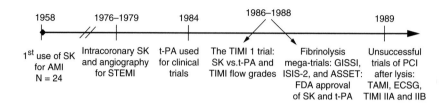

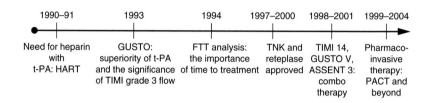

Figure 2.1   Selected highlights from 5 decades of fibrinoloysis

II.   EARLY HISTORY, 1958

The first report of the use of a thrombolytic agent to treat acute myocardial infarction was published in 1958 (1). Tony Fletcher and Sol Sherry, then at the Washington University School of Medicine in St. Louis, treated 24 patients with relatively prolonged ($\leq$30 hours) and high-dose (35–100,000 U/h) intravenous (iv) infusions of streptokinase (SK) during evolving AMI. The paper would not have been accepted for publication by today's standards for a number of reasons: the patient selection criteria were not defined, the dose and duration of SK varied widely and with no reported rationale, and there were no prespecified endpoints. Nevertheless, the account is seminal for presenting several concepts that proved to be of tremendous importance over ensuing decades:

1.   The idea that pharmacological dissolution of an occlusive coronary artery thrombus could result in myocardial salvage, with a smaller area of infarction and clinical benefit.
2.   Demonstration of induction of a systemic thrombolytic state in humans (documented by lowering of fibrinogen and plasminogen levels).

3. Demonstration of faster washout of cardiac enzyme (SGOT) than usually observed.
4. Demonstration that administration of SK results in prolongation of the prothrombin time (PT).
5. Speculation on the importance of time to treatment—patients were divided into an early treatment group (6–14 h) and a delayed treatment group (20–72 h).
6. Speculation on the importance of anticoagulation therapy after thrombolytic therapy.
7. Speculation on the relative safety of such therapy (albeit in a very small number of patients).

Although this study demonstrated the logic and feasibility of thrombolytic therapy for acute AMI, its impact was minimal due to the very small sample size and the lack of angiographic or any other conclusive endpoints. Although there was some ongoing interest in the concept, especially in Europe, real progress was not made for another two decades.

III. THE BEGINNING OF THE MODERN ERA, 1979–1980

The modern thrombolytic era began in 1979, when three important observations came together. Marcus DeWood and colleagues in Spokane were interested in emergency coronary artery bypass surgery for evolving AMI (2). In order to accomplish this, patients had to undergo emergency cardiac catheterization and coronary angiography. Previously, AMI was considered a contraindication to coronary angiography: it was felt that administration of contrast agent would result in hemodynamic instability and/or the induction of intractable dysrhythmias. (The contrast agents available in the 1970s had profound negative inotropic and chronotropic effects.) This study demonstrated the relative safety of angiography during evolving MI. More important, a very high rate of coronary artery obstruction due to intraluminal thrombus was demonstrated. This was the first documentation that intracoronary thrombosis was the proximate cause of coronary artery obstruction leading to AMI and not a secondary or postmortem event, as had been postulated by many pathologists. Furthermore, the patients undergoing angiography at the earliest time points after symptom onset had the highest rate of thrombosis, presumably due to spontaneous thrombolysis from endogenous plasmin activation occurring in those studied later.

The third observation that precipitated a surge of interest in thrombolytic therapy was the angiographic demonstration by Peter Rentrop and colleagues of the dissolution of intracoronary thrombus by the direct intracoronary administration of streptokinase in 1979 (3). [This had previously been reported by Chazov et al. in 1976, but the report was in Russian and escaped the attention of western cardiologists (4).] The largely unsuccessful efforts during the 1970s to reduce the size of myocardial infarction by decreasing myocardial oxygen demand were suddenly supplanted by a spate of preclinical and clinical studies to determine whether thrombolysis could be induced quickly enough and safely enough to produce clinically significant reductions of infarct size by increasing oxygen supply through restoration of coronary blood flow.

IV. ANGIOGRAPHIC ASSESSMENT

The early clinical studies of thrombolysis were performed in the cardiac catheterization suite for several reasons. Initially, a guidewire was advanced into the thrombus to mechanically disrupt it and increase the area exposed to the thrombolytic drug. In some cases, a small catheter was advanced to the proximal surface of the clot in order to more directly administer the drug. This was felt to be especially important when there were large coronary branches proximal to the clotted segment. Intracoronary or subselective injection was thought to be more likely to be successful than systemic intravenous therapy because of the ability to provide relatively high local concentrations of drug. This turned out to be true for streptokinase but not for more fibrin-specific drugs. It was also hoped that the induction of a systemic lytic state could be avoided by giving lower doses of streptokinase locally. This actually was not the case, because the doses employed for intracoronary treatment were high enough (generally >150,000 units of streptokinase) such that profound systemic fibrinolysis was usually observed. However, recanalization trials required the angiographic demonstration of intra-coronary thrombus prior to the administration of the thrombolytic drug, whether it be by the intracoronary or the systemic route. Subsequent angiography could then demonstrate both the time course and success rate of the thrombolytic regimen studied.

Efforts to decrease the time until therapy was initiated to maxi-mize both the rate of success of lytic therapy [fresher clots are more susceptible to lysis, especially with nonfibrin-specific agents (5)] and the impact of reperfusion on myocardial salvage led to a shift to intra-venous administration of these drugs, which could be performed in the coronary care unit (CCU) or the emergency department (ED), saving 1–2 hours between diagnosis and the initiation of therapy. Trials per-formed with angiographic assessment after the initiation of throm-bolytic therapy are patency studies: infarct-related vessels found to be patent will include those that contained clot that was successfully dissolved by the therapy delivered, those that contained clot that resolved because of the body's own fibrinolytic mechanisms before therapy was instituted, and those that never had intracoronary thrombus as an occlusive event.

Recanalization trials in which serial angiography was performed at 10- to 15-minute intervals have consistently demonstrated an S-shaped curve of achieving flow restoration (6). In some patients normal flow is observed within 15 minutes of starting therapy, a few more will have open vessels at 30 minutes, and even more at 45 minutes. While increased patency may be observed out to 24 hours, successful throm-bolysis is generally defined as restoration of flow within 90 minutes. This has been accepted as a standard endpoint for several reasons. It is a short enough interval to expect a benefit from reperfusion. For recanalization studies in the catheterization laboratory, it is at about the level of endurance of both the patient and the operator. In patency trials, especially early studies, 90 minutes was the usual interval from the start of therapy until the first angiogram could be performed. Given the notorious insensitivity and unreliability of noninvasive markers of rep-erfusion, angiography has remained the gold standard for assessing thrombolytic regimens in pilot studies of ~50 to a few hundred patients, with mortality the preferred endpoint in large clinical trials.

V. RECOMBINANT t-PA, 1984

Recombinant tissue-type plasminogen activator (t-PA) became available for clinical trials in early 1984. The naturally occurring t-PA molecule had shown promise in a handful of patients treated during acute evolving MI, with six of seven patients having angiographically demonstrated thrombolysis within 20–50 minutes of initiation of therapy (7). The recombinant form of this molecule could be produced in sufficient quantities to treat any number of patients with whatever dose was required. In the pilot study of recombinant t-PA, 75% (25/33) of patients treated with 0.5–0.75 mg/kg of t-PA iv over 30–120 minutes exhibited recanalization within 90 minutes. Only one of the 14 control patients exhibited recanalization during this observation period. The remaining 13 control patients were subsequently crossed over to be treated with t-PA 0.375 mg/kg by the intracoronary route over 15–30 minutes. Of these, 69% (9/13) exhibited recanalization within 45 minutes (8).

VI. THE TIMI I TRIAL, 1987

The Thrombolysis in Myocardial Infarction (TIMI) trials have become a series of National Institutes of Health (NIH)-sponsored studies, largely under the direction of Eugene Braunwald, looking at various aspects of reperfusion therapy for evolving MI. (Twenty-eight TIMI trials had been completed or launched as of late 2003.) The first of these trials was initially conceived as a large clinical study to determine whether thrombolytic therapy of AMI could really have an impact on mortality. However, a debate ensued about which thrombolytic drug to use in the treatment arm of the trial. There was considerable experience by that time with streptokinase. On the other hand, t-PA looked very promising in small angiographic studies and could have supplanted streptokinase as the treatment of choice by the time the trial was completed. However, it was felt that there was not yet enough clinical experience with t-PA to warrant its use in such a large study. Thus, the TIMI I trial evolved into an initial study to directly compare streptokinase and t-PA in a randomized angiographic recanalization study (6).

Table 2.1 TIMI Flow Grades

TIMI 0: No antegrade flow beyond the obstructed site in the infarct-related artery
TIMI 1: Limited antegrade flow, without complete visualization of the infarct-related artery
TIMI 2: Complete, but delayed, filling of the infarct related artery
TIMI 3: Prompt, complete filling of the infarct-related artery, with or without a residual stenosis

In the TIMI I study, 232 patients with evolving AMI presenting within 7 hours of symptom onset were taken immediately to the catheterization suite. After initial angiography-demonstrated thrombotic occlusion, patients were randomized to receive intravenous recombinant t-PA in a dose of 80 mg infused over 3 hours or iv streptokinase in a dose of 1.5 million units infused over 1 hour. At the time, this was a very large dose of streptokinase, but there had been some experience with it and it was felt that any smaller dose might unfairly bias the trial in favor of t-PA. Heparin was also administered intravenously, but aspirin was not given until discharge. Patients were kept in the catheterization lab, and serial angiograms were performed at 15-minute intervals until 90 minutes had passed since the initiation of thrombolytic therapy. The TIMI flow grades, initially developed at Washington University by Tiefenbrunn and Sobel in response to the RFP for TIMI 1 and during initial protocol development, were introduced in this study to describe the degree of flow observed in the epicardial vessels following therapy (Table 2.1). TIMI grade 0 indicated no antegrade flow in the infarct-related artery; grade 1 indicated a trickle of flow but a lack of complete filling; grade 2 indicated delayed but eventual complete visualization of the vessel; and grade 3 indicated normal antegrade flow, with or without a residual narrowing at the site of recent occlusion.

Twice as many vessels exhibited recanalization with TIMI grade 2 or 3 flow at 90 minutes following the administration of t-PA compared to those receiving streptokinase (62 vs. 31%; $p < 0.01$). In addition, recanalization was observed earlier in the patients receiving t-PA. It was also observed that streptokinase exhibited decreased efficacy in patients treated later, i.e., with presumably older, more organized thrombi, while this difference was not evident in those receiving t-PA.

VII.   MORTALITY TRIALS, 1986–1988

Three relatively large randomized clinical trials of thrombolytic therapy for AMI were completed in the mid-1980s. The first of these was the GISSI trial, performed in Italy (9). In this study, 11,712 patients with evolving AMI were randomized to receive streptokinase or not (no placebo was given). Treatment had to be initiated within 12 hours of symptom onset. Mortality at 30 days was reduced by 18%, from 13.0 to 10.7%. Patients treated within 1 hour had a remarkable mortality reduction of 47%. Heparin and aspirin therapies were not specified in this trial. Very few patients (< 3%) underwent angioplasty or coronary artery bypass grafting surgery (CABG) during their initial hospitalization, but the survival curves for the treated and untreated patients remained parallel during subsequent 1-year follow-up observation (10).

The second study was the European International Study of Infarct Survival (ISIS II) Trial (11). This study randomized patients suspected of having an AMI (there were no ECG inclusion criteria) to one of four arms: placebo, aspirin only, streptokinase only, or streptokinase plus aspirin. Thus, this was the first large trial of combination therapy to evaluate the impact of treating both the fibrin and the platelet components of clot. Of 17,187 patients randomized, mortality at 30 days was lowered by 21% in those treated with streptokinase, from 13.2% in the placebo group to 10.4%, with a similar 19% reduction to 10.7% in those treated with aspirin alone. Those receiving both agents had a 39% reduction in mortality to 8.0% ($p < 0.05$ for all comparisons). These patients were enrolled up to 24 hours after symptom onset, and the median time to treatment was 5 hours. Heparin therapy was not included in the protocol regimen.

The third large trial was the Anglo Scandinavian Study of Early Thrombolysis (ASSET) (12). In this study, 5011 patients with AMI presenting within 5 hours were randomized to receive placebo or t-PA 100 mg infused over 3 hours. Mortality at 30 days was reduced by 27% in those receiving t-PA, from 9.8 to 7.2%. Heparin was given, but aspirin was not included in the treatment protocol.

These three large trials, in combination with a number of smaller randomized controlled studies, firmly established the ability of early thrombolytic therapy to favorably impact outcome in patients with evolving AMI.

VIII. FDA APPROVAL, 1987–1989

Streptokinase was first used in humans in the 1940s by direct infusion into the thoracic cavity to help lyse pleural adhesions. This was the agent given intravenously in the 1950s in the first attempts to treat acute myocardial infarction, and it was the agent used in the early attempts at intracoronary therapy for thrombolysis. Streptokinase is a bacterial protein that combines with plasminogen in the circulation to form a streptokinase-plasminogen complex that acts as an activator of other plasminogen molecules to the proteolytic enzyme plasmin. Plasmin in turn works to dissolve fibrin clot as well as circulating fibrinogen. This agent was approved by the U.S. Food and Drug Administration (FDA) in late 1987 for the intravenous therapy of AMI.

t-PA is a human protein initially isolated from a melanoma cell line by Desire Collen (7). The molecule was subsequently cloned and produced by recombinant DNA technology in a mammalian cell line by Genentech, Inc. t-PA is a direct plasminogen activator that is fibrin specific, that is, it binds preferentially to fibrin and fibrin-bound plasminogen, resulting in minimal activation of circulating plasminogen and minimal fibrinogenolysis in therapeutic doses. Fibrin specificity itself results in improved efficacy, plus it helps to avoid depletion of circulating plasminogen, which can limit the efficacy of nonfibrin-specific agents, especially when given in high doses (13). Furthermore, as a human protein, t-PA is not allergenic. This agent was approved by FDA in December 1987.

Anisolated plasminogen streptokinase activator complex (APSAC) is a time-released form of streptokinase. A streptokinase-plasminogen complex is formed in vitro and then acylated. This was the first agent designed to be administered as an intravenous bolus. The molecule does not activate plasminogen to plasmin until undergoing chemical deacylation in the circulation. This agent was approved by FDA in 1989. The primary attraction of APSAC is the ability to administer this agent as a single intravenous bolus. However, its efficacy is similar to that of streptokinase, with a dollar cost similar to t-PA, and its use was never widespread and is currently rare (<1% of patients treated in the United States).

IX. ADJUNCTIVE ANGIOPLASTY AFTER THROMBOLYSIS, 1987–1989

In the pioneering studies of thrombolytic therapy for AMI there was great concern about the issue of reocclusion. It was known that all of the thrombolytic drugs produced at least some degree of plasminemia and that plasmin activated thrombin. Thus, a procoagulant state was being induced at the same time that thrombus was being dissolved. In addition, the ruptured plaque that initially led to thrombosis was still there and represented a nidus for recurrent thrombosis until reendotheliation occurred. Although more recent studies have consistently demonstrated angiographic reocclusion rates of 5–6% with corresponding clinical reinfarction rates of 2.5–3%, early estimates of the rate of reocclusion were high, in the range of 30%, and it was known that reocclusion was associated with high mortality (14). Reocclusion was also felt to be more likely to occur in the presence of a high-grade residual stenosis after clot resolution.

Three studies were undertaken to determine whether angioplasty of infarct-related arteries early after successful thrombolysis would be beneficial in preventing early reocclusion and therefore improve survival and left ventricular function. The first of these was the Thrombolysis and Angioplasty in Acute Myocardial Infarction (TAMI I) trial, led by Eric Topol (15). In this study, 386 patients with AMI treated with t-PA were taken immediately (within 2 hours of starting thrombolytic treatment) to the catheterization laboratory. Patients with a patent-infarct-related artery with an underlying stenosis suitable for PCI (about half of the total) were randomized to immediate PCI or conservative management, with a follow-up angiogram 1 week later in all patients. Of those in the conservative group, 16% subsequently required PCI and 2% underwent bypass surgery because of recurrent ischemia. Reocclusion rates and mortality were identical in the two groups, but transfusion requirements and emergency bypass surgery rates were higher in those patients with immediate PCI. It is of note that 14% of the conservatively managed patients did not have a hemodynamically significant residual stenosis at the 1-week follow-up angiogram.

The TIMI IIA study was of similar design and randomized 392 patients (16). The incidence of reocclusion was not reduced, but complication rates were higher in those patients undergoing immediate PCI. Patency at 1 week was high, whether patients underwent early PCI or conservative management, averaging 84%. A third study sponsored by the European Cooperative Study Group used a similar design, randomizing 367 patients (17). Once again, there was no apparent benefit to emergency PCI, but there was a twofold increase in the rate of adverse events.

A fourth study, TIMI IIB, asked a somewhat different question (18). If emergency PCI after successful thrombolysis is not necessary, is it still important to perform angiography and possibly PCI routinely 18–48 hours after pharmacological therapy? (There was also a delayed invasive therapy group of 194 patients in the TIMI IIA trial.) In TIMI IIB, 3339 patients with AMI were treated with t-PA (3-hour infusion), aspirin, iv heparin, and β-blocker, if not contraindicated. They were randomized to protocol-mandated angiography at 18–48 hours, with PCI if appropriate, or conservative management with angiography performed only if indicated by recurrent ischemic symptoms or a positive stress study. In the 6 weeks following randomization, approximately 25% of the conservatively managed group had undergone PCI or bypass surgery. Revascularization was performed in 66% of those in the invasive group. In spite of this high rate of revascularization, the incidence of recurrent MI (6.1%) and death (5.0%) was identical in the two groups. Survival and left ventricular ejection fraction at one year were also not significantly different.

Thus, neither emergency nor elective cardiac catheterization and PCI have been shown to be necessary to consolidate the gains of successful reperfusion in patients who are doing well clinically, a finding presaged by the stable course of patients after thrombolysis in trials such as GISSI, in which subsequent revascularization was rare.

It should be kept in mind that the angioplasty equipment available in the 1980s when the above studies were performed was still relatively primitive. Not only were stents not available to treat dissections, but deflated balloons were bulky and relatively inflexible. Visualization of the vessel being worked on was virtually impossible when the balloon catheter was deployed across the lesion, even with injections through both the guide catheter and the balloon catheter lumen. At that time, trans stenotic pressure gradients were still being measured to assess success. There were no debulking techniques or distal protection devices, and glycoprotein IIb/IIIa inhibiting agents were not yet clinically available.

X. ACCELERATED T-PA, 1989

Early-dose regimens of t-PA were based on two premises: its relatively short half-life in the circulation (actually multicompartmented, but usually expressed as approximately 5 minutes) and the need to "bathe" the offending thrombus in lytic long enough to achieve complete clot dissolution and minimize the risk of thrombotic reocclusion. An initial bolus was not originally employed because the time to achieve equilibrium in the circulation was so brief because of the short half-life. Duration of infusion extended to as long as 6 hours in some trials. The FDA-approved regimen was a 3-hour infusion, with a standard dose of 100 mg given as 40 mg over the first hour and then 30 mg per hour for the next 2 hours. In 1989 Karl Neuhaus reported an accelerated or "front-loaded" regimen in which t-PA was given as a 15-mg bolus followed by an additional 35 mg over 30 minutes (half of the total dose within 30 min), with the last 50 mg infused over 60 minutes (total dose within 90 min). In 74 patients treated with this regimen, 91% exhibited patency (TIMI 2 or 3 flow) within 90 minutes (19). The success of this regimen is predicated on two factors. Although the half-life of t-PA in the circulation is very short, it has been documented that t-PA binds to the fibrin clot and lytic activity can persist for hours (20). Thus, high initial levels can result in higher adsorption to the clot and jump-start the lytic process. However, the relatively brief exposure to high levels of t-PA does not result in the elevated bleeding complications that were observed when the total dose was increased (21). Reocclusion is minimized by prompt conjuctive therapy with aspirin and heparin.

XI. GISSI II AND THE INTERNATIONAL T-PA/SK MORTALITY TRIAL, 1990

As one of the first recombinant DNA products to reach the marketplace, t-PA was expensive to develop and produce and was priced at a relatively high level ($2,200 when it was introduced in 1987, with no subsequent increase or decrease), approximately five times the cost of treating a patient with streptokinase. Thus, even though there was convincing angiographic evidence of its superiority to streptokinase in producing higher rates of reperfusion and faster reperfusion, there was considerable impetus to demonstrate that these angiographic findings could be translated into a measurable and significant difference in clinical outcome.

This issue was addressed by two coordinated European trials, GISSI II and the the International t-PA/SK Mortality Trial (22,23). The combined studies included nearly 21,000 patients with AMI who were randomized to receive SK 1.5 million units over 1 hour or t-PA 100 mg over 3 hours. Some patients received late (>12 h) subcutaneous heparin, but no iv heparin was used. Mortality at 2 weeks was not different in those receiving t-PA compared to SK (8.9 vs. 8.5%, respectively; $p = $ NS). With subsequent documentation of the importance of iv heparin in patients treated with t-PA (see below), it became clear that the lack of a difference in mortality in this trial, and the relatively high mortality observed, was likely related to inadequate conjunctive antithrombin therapy in those patients receiving t-PA.

XII. IMPORTANCE OF CONJUNCTIVE ANTITHROMBIN THERAPY, 1991

Most cardiologists were so convinced that a period of anti thrombin therapy after administration of a thrombolytic drug was necessary that nobody bothered to perform a controlled clinical trial to address this issue until the early 1990s (24). Two relatively small but pivotal angiographic studies were performed to assess this question. The first of these was the Heparin or Aspirin Reocclusion Trial (HART), headed by Allan Ross, in which 205 patients were randomized to receive intravenous heparin or not following treatment with t-PA and aspirin for AMI (25). Angiography performed the next day (18–48 hours after initial therapy) demonstrated a significantly higher patency rate in those receiving heparin (82 vs. 52% without heparin; $p < 0.05$). Furthermore, patients who had a consistently therapeutic PTT had a patency rate of 95%, compared to 50% in those in whom PTT were subtherapeutic. A similar trial by Bleich et al. of 160 patients also demonstrated higher patency with heparin at a mean time interval of 48 hours (71 vs. 44%; $p < 0.05$) (26). The more recent HART II trial demonstrated that low molecular weight heparin (enoxaparin) was at least as good as unfractionated heparin as conjunctive therapy in terms of early patency, with a trend toward less reocclusion at 5–7 days in patients treated with enoxaparin (5.9 vs. 9.8%; $p = 0.12$) (27).

XIII. GUSTO: IMPORTANCE OF FULL FLOW RESTORATION

With the failure of GISSI II and the International t-PA/SK Mortality Trial to show a clinical benefit of t-PA relative to SK and with the increased understanding of the importance of a period of antithrombin therapy in conjunction with thrombolysis, at least when a fibrin-specific agent was being used, another large international trial was undertaken, the first GUSTO study (28). In this trial, led by Topol and Califf, more than 40,000 patients presenting within 6 hours of onset of symptoms of AMI were randomized to one of four treatment arms:

1. Accelerated (90-minute infusion) t-PA with adjunctive iv heparin for 48 hours
2. SK 1.5 million units iv (60-minute infusion) with iv heparin
3. SK 1.5 million units iv (60-minute infusion) with subcutaneous (sc) heparin
4. Combined t-PA and SK, each in a reduced dose, followed by iv heparin

All patients received aspirin. The primary endpoint of the trial was mortality at 30 days. There was also an associated angiographic substudy in which a percentage of the patients entered in the clinical trial underwent angiography at various intervals (29).

There was no difference in mortality in patients receiving SK, whether they were treated with iv or sc heparin (7.3 vs. 7.3% at 30 days; p = NS), reinforcing the concept that potent antithrombin therapy is not necessary when the anticoagulant effects of a systemic lytic state are present. Mortality was significantly lower in patients receiving t-PA relative to SK (6.3 vs. 7.3% at 30 days; $p < 0.01$), a relative decrease of 14%. A statistically significant lower mortality following administration of t-PA was evident at 24 hours (2.4 vs. 2.9%; $p < 0.03$). The mortality difference was maintained at 1 year (9.1 vs. 10.1%; $p < 0.02$) (30). The intracranial bleed rate was 0.7% in patients receiving t-PA compared to 0.6% in those treated with SK plus iv heparin (p = NS) and 0.5% in those treated with SK plus sc heparin ($p < 0.02$). The combined endpoint of mortality plus nonfatal stroke ("net clinical benefit") was 7.2, 8.2, and 8.0%, respectively (all comparisons with t-PA have $p < 0.05$).

The reason for the improved mortality following treatment with t-PA was evident from the angiographic substudy, which demonstrated significantly higher rates of TIMI 3 and TIMI 2 + 3 flow at 90 minutes after initiation of therapy with t-PA compared to SK (TIMI 3, 55 vs. 29%; $p < 0.01$; TIMI 2 or 3, 81 vs. 57%; $p < 0.01$). Even though TIMI flow was comparable at 24 hours in patients treated with t-PA or SK, this "catch-up" in patients receiving SK was not of clinical importance; it is only the early restoration of coronary flow that correlated with improved mortality outcome.

The GUSTO trial was the first large study to correlate 90-minute angiographic assessment of TIMI flow grade with the clinical endpoint of mortality at 30 days. There was no difference in mortality for patients exhibiting TIMI 0 compared to TIMI 1 flow, and these patients had the highest mortality, at 8.2%. The lowest mortality, 4.2%, was observed in patients exhibiting TIMI 3 flow. Those with TIMI 2 flow had an intermediate mortality of 7.4%. Subsequent studies have increased the number of patients available for analysis and yielded highly significant differences in mortality of 9.3, 6.1, and 3.7% for patients with TIMI flow rates of 0 or 1, 2, and 3, respectively (31). Patients with TIMI 2 flow represent a mix. This is the most subjective of the grades to assign, although some increase in precision may be obtained by actually counting the number of frames until a vessel is fully visualized (32). Some of these patients will exhibit TIMI 3 flow at a later point in time; some will have reoccluded later (TIMI 0 or 1). Some have actually achieved complete thrombolysis and restoration of flow in the epicardial vessel, but reperfusion was late and distal microvascular reperfusion does not occur because of tissue damage and edema ("no-reflow" phenomenon). It has been observed that even patients with TIMI 3 flow can be subdivided into different "perfusion grades," assessed by the degree of contrast blush evident at angiography, with those exhibiting the best perfusion found to have the lowest mortality (33).

XIV. IMPORTANCE OF TIME TO TREATMENT, 1994

The time dependence of progression of reversible myocardial ischemia to irreversible myocardial infarction is intuitive. Coronary vessels are in general end arteries, and the heart never rests. The onset of physiological changes within minutes of loss of normal blood flow was demonstrated in the 1930s (34). The time course of myocardial infarction in dogs was well outlined by Reimer et al. in the 1970s, with virtually no reversibility evident after 6 hours of persistent ischemia (35). In the early 1980s, Bergman et al. demonstrated a similar time course in dogs with copper coil–induced coronary thrombosis treated with SK (36). The debate has been over what the exact time window is in patients when successful reperfusion can be expected to result in significant myocardial salvage. Initially there was concern that it would not be possible to administer therapy quickly enough to achieve significant salvage in most patients. Subsequently, there was some thought that even very late reperfusion, without demonstrable myocardial salvage, could be of some benefit through improved healing and "remodeling" and decreased tendency to arrhythmias. The earliest randomized trials showed that there was more to be gained in patients treated more quickly, even though there was still measurable benefit in those treated later. The best assessment of the clinically important time frame is the 1994 Fibrinolytic Therapy Trialists (FTT) meta-analysis of all of the large (>1000 patients) randomized trials of thrombolytic therapy versus no reperfusion therapy (37). In this analysis, patients treated within the first hour from symptom onset did best, with 35 lives saved per 1000 patients treated. There was a steep drop-off in benefit after the first hour but then a near-linear decrement in benefit from 2 to 24 hours. Beyond 12 hours, the benefit was relatively small and, in most patients, it was not offset by the risk of therapy. These findings are consistent with the results of the GUSTO trial discussed above. One large randomized trial, the Late Assessment of Thrombolytic Efficacy (LATE) study, also looked at this issue and concluded that initiation of therapy out to 12 hours had potential benefit, again with the caveat that patients treated within the first 1–3 hours have the most to gain (38).

Of course, individual patients may vary widely in how long ischemia might be endured before progressing to infarction. Those with high oxygen demands, e.g., with tachycardia or hypertension, may have a shorter time to irreversible infarction, whereas patients who have developed collateral flow or ischemic preconditioning or who have incomplete or intermittent coronary obstruction may tolerate ischemia for prolonged periods without progressing to infarction of the entire area that is in jeopardy.

Improved understanding of the quantitative impact of treatment delays led to renewed efforts to systematically decrease time to treatment through national programs such as the National Registry of Myocardial Infarction (NRMI), sponsored by Genentech, Inc., and the National Heart Attack Alert Program, sponsored by the National Institute of Health (NIH), which set the goal of treating patients with AMI with a thrombolytic within 30 minutes (39, 40). The median time to treatment for thrombolytic therapy for AMI in patients enrolled in NRMI has decreased from more than 1 hour in 1991 to 33 minutes in 2003. A recent study of more than 27,000 patients from NRMI treated with PCI for AMI demonstrated the importance of prompt therapy in these patients as well, with a significant increase in odds of in-hospital death in those with a door-to-balloon time of greater than 2 hours (41).

XV. IMPORTANCE OF ECG CRITERIA, 1994

The FTT meta-analysis confirmed that it is only patients exhibiting ST segment elevation or a left bundle branch block (LBBB) on the ECG when they present with symptoms of AMI who consistently benefit from thrombolytic therapy. It is not that a patient with thrombotic coronary artery occlusion who has a normal or nonspecific ECG will not benefit from successful reperfusion; it is more the fact that a group of patients with symptoms consistent with myocardial ischemia but with a normal or nonspecific ECG will have a low incidence of occlusion of a major coronary artery, and therefore it would be very difficult to clinically demonstrate benefit of a reperfusion regimen. This is also why trials of different reperfusion regimens generally require strict ECG criteria and treatment within 6 hours, so the impact of treatment is likely to be significant and measurable.

XVI. NEW AGENTS, 1997–2000

Multiple agents for inducing thrombolysis in humans have been explored, including urokinase, pro-urokinase, and the bacterial protein staphylokinase. However, the most promising products and the only category to be brought to market as third-generation thrombolytic drugs are proteins that are modifications of the naturally occurring t-PA molecule. Physiologically, t-PA prevents excessive clot proliferation that could be deleterious and removes clot that is no longer required for hemostasis. Its pharmacodynamic and pharmacokinetic properties are perfect for this role. However, as a pharmaceutical agent used to promote rapid dissolution of relatively large clot burdens, the natural protein offered opportunities for improvement.

One of these agents is reteplase, a deletion mutant of t-PA produced by recombinant DNA technology in *E. coli*. This molecule is not glycosolated (sugars attached to the protein after its manufacture largely determine hepatic uptake and therefore half-life) and has a longer half-life than naturally occurring t-PA. It is administered as two intravenous boluses separated by 30 minutes. It is more fibrin specific than streptokinase but much less fibrin specific than t-PA. In the European INJECT trial, reteplase was compared with streptokinase in a randomized trial of 5936 AMI patients presenting within 6 hours of symptom onset (42). Mortality at 35 days and 6 months was statistically the same for these two agents (8.9 vs. 9.4% at 35 days, 11.0 vs. 12.1% at 6 months for reteplase and streptokinase, respectively; $p = $ NS). The intracranial bleeding (ICB) rate was higher for patients receiving reteplase (0.8 vs. 0.4%; $p < 0.04$), but there was no significant difference in the combined endpoint of 35-day death or nonfatal stroke (9.6 vs. 10.2%; p = NS). The FDA approved reteplase for the treatment of AMI in 1997.

In the RAPID II study, an angiographic patency trial of 303 patients with evolving AMI, reteplase was compared with accelerated (90-min)-dose t-PA (43). The 90-minute TIMI 3 flow rate for patients receiving t-PA was relatively low (compared with that in other similar trials) at 45%, with a significantly higher rate of 60% for those patients treated with reteplase ($p < 0.01$). Based largely on this study, the GUSTO III trial was undertaken to determine whether administration of reteplase to a large number of patients with AMI would be associated with a lower mortality than that observed in patients given t-PA (44). In this trial, patients presenting with AMI within 6 hours were randomized 2:1 to receive double bolus reteplase or t-PA in a weight-adjusted accelerated (90-min) infusion. All patients also received aspirin and intravenous heparin. The 10,138 patients randomized to reteplase had a 30-day mortality of 7.47%, compared to 7.24% for the 4921 patients receiving t-PA (p = NS). Not only was reteplase not demonstrated to be superior to t-PA in terms of mortality, it was felt by the authors that, in spite of the similar numbers, it could not be considered equivalent to t-PA since the confidence limits in this study overlapped the 1% absolute difference in mortality observed in the GUSTO I trial that demonstrated the superiority of t-PA relative to streptokinase. This trial demonstrated a trend to higher relative mortality in patients treated later with reteplase, consistent with the previously observed decreased efficacy in achieving lysis of older clots with nonfibrin-specific agents (6).

The other new product is TNK, developed by Genentech, Inc., as a successor to t-PA. This is not a deletion mutant. It is the result of amino acid substitutions at three different sites along the naturally occurring t-PA molecule; two of these are single substitutions and one is the replacement of one amino acid with a tetra-alanine group. (T, N, and K refer to the single letter abbreviations for the amino acids that were replaced.) The resulting molecule is different from native t-PA in three respects. It is glycosylated differently, resulting in a prolonged half-life of approximately 25 minutes, and it can therefore be administered as a single intravenous bolus. It is even more fibrin specific than t-PA, and it has increased resistance to plasminogen activator inhibitor (45). The results of administration of TNK were evaluated angiographically in the TIMI 10B dose ranging study (46). This trial demonstrated patency rates after a single bolus of 40- or 50-mg TNK that were comparable to those observed with the 90-minute regimen of t-PA. When patients' weights were taken into account, it was found that increasing the dose above 0.5 mg/kg was not associated with increased efficacy but was associated with increased bleeding. Thus, this agent is given on a weight-adjusted basis.

In the ASSENT 2 trial, single-bolus, weight-adjusted TNK was compared with the weight-adjusted accelerated (90-min) t-PA regimen in combination with aspirin and intravenous heparin in 16,505 patients with AMI presenting within 6 hours of symptom onset (47). Mortality at 30 days, intracranial bleed rates, and mortality plus nonfatal stroke rates were virtually identical for the two regimens (6.2 vs. 6.2%, 0.9 vs. 0.9%, and 7.1 vs. 7.2%, respectively; $p = NS$). There was somewhat less (nonintracranial) bleeding with TNK, especially in higher-risk patients (elderly, female, low body weight). Thus, this much simpler to administer drug was found to be equivalent to the established, but relatively complex, t-PA regimen in terms of mortality, with, if anything, a better side effect profile. TNK was approved by the FDA in 2000.

XVII. COMBINED PHARMACOLOGIC THERAPY, 1998–2001

The concept of a two-pronged attack on thrombus by giving a thrombolytic agent to dissolve the fibrin clot and an antiplatelet agent to disrupt the platelet component is not recent—aspirin combined with streptokinase was used successfully in the ISIS II trial published in 1988 and discussed previously. What is new is the availability of the glycoprotein IIb/IIIa–inhibiting agents that block the final common pathway of platelet aggregation and provide much more potent antiplatelet therapy than aspirin. The question is whether adding one of these potent compounds to a thrombolytic could be used to improve the efficacy of reperfusion and/or shorten the time to reperfusion with an acceptable safety profile.

A number of angiographic studies were performed in the late 1990s to address this issue. Perhaps the most comprehensive of these is the TIMI 14 trial, headed by Antman (48). This study enrolled patients with evolving AMI and had two control arms: t-PA alone or abciximab alone. There were multiple treatment arms employing various reduced doses of either t-PA or streptokinase in combination with full-dose abciximab. Heparin was given iv as conjunctive therapy, but in a reduced dose in those receiving abciximab. Angiography was performed within 90 minutes of initiation of treatment. The most promising of these regimens was a half dose of t-PA given over 60 minutes combined with full-dose abciximab, which resulted in a 90-minute TIMI flow grade 3 of 77%, compared with 57% with t-PA alone and 32% with abciximab alone ($p < 0.05$ for both comparisons). However, it should be noted that the number of patients in each subgroup was relatively small (87 patients received the half t-PA + abiximab regimen), and no conclusions regarding safety could be made from this study.

Two large clinical trials evaluated this combined approach. The first of these was the GUSTO V trial (49), in which 16,588 patients with AMI were randomized to receive either reteplase at a standard dose of 10 units iv bolus followed by a second 10-unit bolus after 30 minutes, or 5 units plus 5 units combined with abciximab in a dose of 0.25 mg/kg bolus and 0.125 µg/kg/min iv (maximum 10 µg/min) for 12 hours. All patients were also treated with iv or oral aspirin. The primary endpoint was 30-day mortality, which was not different for the two groups (5.9% with reteplase, 5.6% with combined therapy; $p = $ NS). There was a low absolute reinfarction rate for both groups, but it was significantly lower for those patients receiving the combined regimen (2.3 vs. 3.5%; $p < 0.01$). Unfortunately, bleeding was a serious problem for patients treated with both drugs, with nearly a fourth of these patients (24.6%) having at least minor bleeding and 4.6% having moderate or severe bleeding, compared with 13.7% and 2.3%, respectively, with reteplase alone ($p < 0.05$). Intracranial bleeding was also nearly twice as high in patients over the age of 75 treated with the combined regimen (2.1 vs. 1.1%; $p = .07$).

The second of these trials is the ASSENT 3 study (50). This trial of 6095 patients with AMI had three treatment arms:

1. Full-dose weight-adjusted TNK plus unfractionated heparin
2. Full-dose weight-adjusted TNK plus low molecular weight heparin (enoxaparin)
3. Half-dose weight-adjusted TNK plus abciximab plus unfractionated heparin

Unfractionated heparin was weight adjusted. The abciximab dose was the same regimen used in GUSTO V. Enoxaparin was given as an iv bolus of 30 mg, followed immediately by the first sc dose of 1 mg/kg, which was continued every 12 hours until mechanical revascularization, hospital discharge, or 7 days. All patients received oral aspirin.

This trial was not large enough to use mortality alone as a meaningful endpoint. The primary endpoint was the 30-day incidence of major adverse cardiac events (MACE) (mortality + reinfarction + recurrent ischemia). The lowest incidence of MACE was observed in those patients receiving TNK plus abciximab, 11.1%, compared with 15.4% in the TNK plus unfractionated heparin control group ($p < 0.01$). However, this was offset by a near doubling of the rate of major bleeding from 2.2 to 4.3% ($p < 0.01$). The best overall regimen in this study appeared to be full-dose TNK combined with enoxaparin, which was associated with a significantly lower MACE rate (11.4%; $p < 0.01$ vs. TNK plus unfractionated heparin) with a nonsignificant increase in major bleeding from 2.2 to 3.0%.

The complexity of these regimens, the high dollar cost, and the high bleeding rates observed in these trials have resulted in limited clinical application of thrombolytic plus glycoprotein IIb/IIIa combination therapy. The standard of care for pharmacological reperfusion therapy remains a thrombolytic agent plus conjunctive therapy with aspirin and an antithrombin agent. Adjunctive therapy with a β-blocker and/or a vasodilator when appropriate should be employed using the same criteria as for patients not receiving a reperfusion regimen (51).

Is there an upper limit for the success of thrombolytics in achieving reperfusion? No doubt there is, for several reasons. Not all occlusions are related primarily to thrombosis. Some are due mainly to obstruction by atheromatous material. In some patients the occlusive thrombus may not be readily accessible to systemic therapy because of diffuse and/or severe disease proximally. In some, especially those with ectatic vessels or thrombotically occluded saphenous vein grafts, the clot may be too massive to undergo prompt lysis. The question really is not whether there is a "ceiling," but how high it is. Even with combined regimens that push the limits of safety, it has been difficult to consistently demonstrate early TIMI 3 flow in more than approximately 75% of treated patients.

XVIII. COMBINED PHARMACOLOGICAL AND MECHANICAL THERAPY, 1999–2003

As successful as thrombolytic therapy has been, it does have several limitations. Early restoration of flow is not observed in at least a quarter of the patients treated. The risk of intracranial bleeding is 0.7–0.9% overall in many large studies but clearly higher in the elderly. Largely because of this risk, patients must meet strict ECG criteria to be considered for treatment. Early mechanical opening of occluded vessels in patients with evolving MI with the use of percutaneous coronary intervention techniques was first reported by Hartzler et al. in 1983 (52). This approach became much more widespread following the 1993 report from the PAMI trial indicating a lower early mortality in patients undergoing PCI compared with those receiving t-PA (53). Increased enthusiasm for this approach correlated with improvements in angioplasty equipment. Patients suspected of MI, but without ECG evidence of ST segment elevation, can be referred for catheterization and possible PCI. The success rate in achieving reperfusion is very high, and since the underlying stenosis is treated at the same time, rates of recurrent MI and recurrent ischemia are generally low. Although conjunctive therapy with an antithrombin agent and, more recently, a glycoprotein IIb/IIIa–inhibiting agent is often used with PCI, intracranial bleeding rates are negligible when compared to lytic therapy. PCI may be especially preferred in patients with AMI complicated by cardiogenic shock, when the thrombolytic may not reach the offending thrombus well because of inadequate perfusion pressure (54). A recent meta-analysis of 23 trials confirmed many cardiologists' conviction that PCI is the preferred approach to acute MI when it is readily available (55).

Availability is the major weakness of the mechanical approach. Performing PCI on acutely ill AMI patients requires a skilled and experienced operator and team. Many hospitals receiving AMI patients do not have catheterization laboratories or such teams. Those that do may have all of their procedure rooms busy during the day, and there may be unacceptable delays in the off hours to assemble the necessary staff. The benefits of PCI, like thrombolysis, are time dependent (41). Unlike thrombolysis, PCI requires a certain volume of patients to develop and maintain operator skills (56,57); therefore, concentrating this approach at specialized centers is attractive.

One approach to the dilemma of treating quickly with a thrombolytic versus more effective but relatively delayed therapy with PCI is planned combined therapy [pharmacoinvasive therapy (58)] with administration of a thrombolytic drug on the way to the catheterization laboratory. This approach has the advantage of prompt initiation of therapy that may be effective in achieving reperfusion in a significant percentage of patients before they can reach a catheterization facility and undergo angiography. In those with delayed, incomplete, or failed thrombolysis, relatively prompt PCI will still be available.

This idea was studied in the Plasminogen Activator Angioplasty Compatibility Trial (PACT) (59). Patients with acute MI were randomized to receive a 50-mg dose of t-PA or placebo on the way to an experienced PCI facility. If early (<1 h) angiography demonstrated TIMI 3 flow in the infarct-related artery, they received a second dose of drug or placebo. All others underwent immediate PCI. The goal of this study was twofold: to determine whether a significant number of patients would respond to lytic treatment before mechanical reperfusion was even an option and to determine whether having been treated with the lytic drug was a detriment to obtaining a good result when PCI needed to be performed. Of the 606 patients randomized, twice as many receiving t-PA had TIMI 2 or 3 flow on the first angiogram compared to placebo (61 vs. 31%; $p < 0.05$). Furthermore, results of PCI were excellent and no different with or without t-PA "on board." Very few patients in this study received stents or a IIb/IIIa inhibitor. Other studies are underway to evaluate different lytic and lytic/glycoprotein IIb/IIIa regimens and different delays to PCI on the impact of this promising therapeutic approach and will be discussed elsewhere in this text.

Table 2.2 FDA-Approved Thrombolytic Agents for Intravenous Use in the Treatment of Acute MI

	Agent				
	SK	TPA	APSAC	RPA	TNK
Proprietary name	Streptase	Activase	Eminase	Retavase	TNKase
Nonproprietary name	Streptokinase	Alteplase	Anistreplase	Reteplase	Tenecteplase
Fibrin specificity	None	High	None	Minimal	Very high
Dosing infusion	60 min	Bolus/ 90 min	Bolus	2 boluses/ 30 min	Bolus
Dosing level	1.5 million units	Max. 100 mg[a]	30 mg.	10 units × 2	Max. 50 mg[a]
Approval date	1987	1987	1989	1997	2000
Company/ Distributor	Aventis/ Behring	Genentech	b	Scios	Genentech

[a] Weight-adjusted dosing.
[b] No longer distributed in the United States; not listed in Physicians' Desk Reference (PDR).

XIX. THE FUTURE

There are ongoing efforts to continue to enhance the benefits of pharmacological reperfusion therapy. New thrombolytic agents are being evaluated. However, the dollar market for these drugs is small by pharmaceutical company standards (although these agents are expensive, most patients are treated only once in their lifetime), and the cost of development and bringing a new drug or biological agent to market may preclude the future availability of a successor to TNK. There is still interest in the potential of combined therapy with a thrombolytic and a potent antiplatelet agent, either a glycoprotein IIb/IIIa inhibitor or a thienopyridine ADP inhibitor such as clopidogrel. Earlier initiation of therapy is still a goal. There are logistic, economic, and legal hurdles to prehospital therapy, especially in the United States, but this approach has the potential for significantly shortening time to treatment, especially in rural areas where ambulance runs are long. Providing early thrombolytic therapy to eligible patients who are being referred for PCI, but in whom a significant delay to mechanical reperfusion is anticipated, shows great promise and is undergoing further investigation. Finally, there are ongoing efforts to improve the benefits of both pharmacological and mechanical reperfusion by augmenting both microvascular and tissue protection within areas of myocardium where flow has been restored.

Even as we continue to evolve better therapeutic approaches to reperfusion therapy in AMI, the most important factor in the short term may be ensuring that as many eligible patients as possible receive this potentially life-saving therapy. In a recent study from the NRMI data base, approximately 25% of patients who met the criteria for thrombolysis and had no apparent contraindications did not receive lytic therapy or primary PCI (60). An even more impressive finding from this study was that it was often the sickest patients who were not treated.

XX. CONCLUSIONS

It is difficult to overestimate the importance of pharmacological reperfusion therapy for evolving AMI. Literally hundreds of thousands of lives have been saved worldwide since this therapy became accepted in the mid-1980s. In terms of the number of patients enrolled in pilot studies, large randomized controlled trials, and registries, no other therapy in the history of medicine has been so thoroughly evaluated. It remains the treatment of choice for patients with AMI when mechanical reperfusion approaches are not readily available. Fortunately, the principles established for pharmacological reperfusion, including the importance of time to treatment, maximizing both epicardial and tissue level perfusion, and providing appropriate conjunctive and adjunctive therapy, have carried over to mechanical reperfusion therapy for AMI.

REFERENCES

1. Fletcher AP, Alkjaersig N, Smyrniotis FE, Sherry S. The treatment of patients suffering from early myocardial infarction with massive and prolonged streptokinase therapy. *Trans Assoc Am Phys. 1958; 71:287–296.*

2. DeWood MA, Spores J, Notske RN, Mouser LT, Burroughs R, Golden MS, Lang HT. Prevalence of total coronary occlusion during the early hours of transmural myocardial infarction. *N Engl J Med. 1980; 303:897–903.*

3. Rentrop P, Blanke H, Karsch KR, Wiegand V, Kostering K, Oster H, Leitz K. Acute myocardial infarction: intracoronary application of nitroglycerin and streptokinase in combination with transluminal recanalization. *Clin Cardiol. 1979; 2:354–363.*

4. Chazov EL, Matteeva LS, Mazaev AV, et al. Intracoronary administration of fibrinolysis in acute myocardial infarction. *Ter Arkh. 1976; 48(4):8–19.*

5. Fox, KAA, Robison AK, Knabb RM, Rosamond TL, Sobel BE, Bergmann SR. Prevention of coronary thrombosis with subthrombolytic doses of tissue-type plasminogen activator. *Circulation 1985; 72:1346–1354.*

6. Chesebro JH, Knatterud G, Roberts R, Borer J, Cohen LS, Dalen J, Dodge HT, Francis CK, Hillis D, Ludbrook PA, Markis JE, Mueller H, Passamani ER, Powers ER, Rao AK, Robertson T, Ross A, Ryan TJ, Sobel, BE, Willerson J, Williams DO, Zaret BL, Braunward E. Thrombolysis in myocardial infarction (TIMI) Trial, Phase I: a comparison between intravenous tissue plasminogen activator and intravenous streptokinase. *Circulation 1987; 76:142–154.*

7. Van de Werf F, Ludbrook PA, Bergmann SR, Tiefenbrunn AJ, Fox KA, de Geest H, Verstraete M, Collen D, Sobel B. Coronary thrombolysis with tissue-type plasminogen activator in patients with evolving myocardial infarction. *N Engl J Med 1984; 310:609–616 (March).*

8. Collen D, Topol EJ, Tiefenbrunn AJ, Gold HK, Weisfeldt ML, Sobel BE, Leinbach RC, Brinker JA, Ludbrook PA, Uasuda I, Bulkley BH, Robinson AK, Hutter AM, Bell WR, Spadaro JJ, Khaw BA, Grossbard EB. Coronary thrombolysis with recombinant human tissue-type plasminogen activator: a prospective randomized, placebo-controlled trial. *Circulation 1984; 70(6):1012–1017.*

9. Gruppo Italiano per lo studio della streptochinasi nell'infarto miocardico (GISSI). Effectiveness of intravenous thrombolytic treatment in acute myocardial infarction. *Lancet 1986; i:397–401.*

10. Gruppo Italiano per lo Studio della streptochinasi nell'infarto miocardico (GISSI). Long term effects of intravenous thrombolysis in acute myocardial infarction: final report of the GISSI study. *Lancet 1987; ii:871–874.*

11. ISIS-2 (second International Study of Infarct Survival) Collaborative Group. Randomised trial of intravenous streptokinase, oral aspirin, both, or neither among 17 187 cases of suspected acute myocardial infarction: ISIS-2. *Lancet 1988; ii:349–360.*

12. Wilcox RG, Von Deer Life G, Olsson CG, Jensen G, Skene AM, Hampton JR, for the Asset Study Group. Trial of tissue plasminogen activator for mortality reduction in acute myocardial infarction. Anglo-Scandinavian Study of Early Thrombolysis (ASSET). *Lancet 1988; ii: 525–530.*

13. Sobel BE, Nachowiak DA, Fry ETA, Bergmann SR, Torr SR. Paradoxical attenuation of fibrinolysis attributable to "plasminogen steal" and its implications for coronary thrombolysis. *Coronary Artery Dis 1991; 1:111–119.*

14. Ohman EM, Califf RM, Topol EJ et al. Consequence of reocclusion after successful reperfusion therapy in acute myocardial infarction: The TAMI Study Group. *Circulation 1990; 82:781–791.*

15. Topol EJ, Califf RM, George BS, Kereiakes DJ, Abbottsmith CW, Candela RJ, Lee KL, Pitt B, Stack RS, O'Neill WW. The thrombolysis and angioplasty in myocardial infarction (TAMI) study group. A multicenter randomized trial of intravenous recombinant tissue plasminogen activator and immediate angioplasty in acute myocardial infarction. *N Eng J Med 1987; 317:581–588.*

16. The TIMI Research Group. Immediate vs. delayed catheterization angioplasty following thrombolytic therapy for acute myocardial infarction. TIMI II A results. *JAMA 1988; 260:2849–2858.*

17. Simoons ML, Arnold AER, Betriu A, de Bono DP, Col J, Dougherty FC, von Essen R, Lambertz H, Lubsen J, Meier B, Michel PL, Raynaud R, Rutsh W, Sanz GA, Schmidt W, Serruys PW, Thery C, Uebis R, Vahanian A, Van De Werf F, Wood D, Verstraete M for the European Cooperative Study Group for Recombinant Tissue-Type Plasminogen Activator in Acute Myocardial Infarction. No additional benefit from immediate percutaneous coronary angioplasty. *Lancet 1988; i:197–202.*

18. The TIMI Study Group. Comparison of invasive and conservative strategies after treatment with intravenous tissue plasminogen activator in acute myocardial infarction. Results of the Thrombolysis in Myocardial Infarction (TIMI) Phase II Trial. *N Engl J Med 1989; 320:618–627.*

19. Neuhaus KL, Feuerer W, Jeep-Tebbe S, Niederer W, Vogt A, Tebbe U. Improved thrombosis with a modified dose regimen of recombinant tissue-type plasminogen activator. *J Am Coll Cardiol 1989; 14:1566–1569.*

20. Eisenberg PR, Sherman LA, Tiefenbrunn AJ, Ludbrook PA, Sobel BE, Jaffe AS. Sustained fibrinolysis after administration of t-PA despite its short half-life in the circulation. *Thrombos Homeostasis 1987; 57(1): 540.*

21. Smalling RW, Schumacher R, Morris D, et al. Improved infarct-related arterial patency after high dose, weight-adjusted, rapid infusion of tissue-type plasminogen activator in myocardial infarction: results of a multicenter randomized trial of two dosage regimens. *J Am Coll Cardiol 1990; 15:912–921.*

22. Gruppo Italiano per Lo Studio Della Sopravvivenza Nell'Infarto Miocardico GISSI-2. A factorial randomized trial of alteplase versus streptokinase and myocardial infarction. *Lancet 1990; 336:65–71.*

23. The International Study Group. In-hospital mortality and clinical course of 20891 patients with suspected acute myocardial infarction randomised between alteplase and streptokinase with or without heparin. *Lancet 1990; 336:71–75.*

24. Sobel BE: Conjunctive therapy for thrombolysis. *Coron Artery Dis 1992, 3:987–989.*

25. Hsia J, Hamilton WP, Kleiman N, Roberts R, Chaitman BR, Ross AN and the HART Investigators. A comparison between heparin and low-dose aspirin as adjunative therapy with tissue plasminogen activator in acute myocardial infarction. *N Engl J Med 1990; 323:1433–1437.*

26. Bleich SD, Nichols T, Schumacher R, et al. Effect of heparin on coronary arterial patency after thrombolysis with tissue plasminogen activator in acute myocardial infarction. *Am J Cardiol 1990; 66:1412–1417.*

27. Ross AM, Molhoek P, Lundergan C, Knudtson M, Draoui Y, Regalado L, Le Louer V, Bigonzi F, Scwartz W, de Jong E, Coyne K. Randomized comparison of enoxaparin, a low-molecular-weight heparin, with unfractionated heparin adjunctive to recombinant tissue plasminogen activator thrombolysis and aspirin. Second trial of heparin and aspirin reperfusion therapy (HART II). *Circulation 2001; 104:648–652.*

28. The GUSTO Investigators. An international randomized trial comparing four thrombolytic strategies for acute myocardial infarction. *N Engl J Med. 1993; 329:673–682.*

29. The GUSTO Angiographic Investigators. The effects of tissue plasminogen activator, streptokinase, or both on coronary-artery patency, ventricular function, and survival after acute myocardial infarction. *N Engl J Med. 1993; 329:1615–1622.*

30. Califf RM, White HD, Van de Werf F, et al. One year results from the global utilization of streptokinase and t-PA for occluded coronary arteries (GUSTO-I) trial. *Circulation 1996; 94:1233–1238.*

31. Gibson CM. Insights into the pathophysiology of acute coronary syndromes using the TIMI flow grade and TIMI frame counting methods. In: Cannon CP, ed. Contemporary Management of Acute Coronary Syndromes. Totowa, NJ: *Humana Press; 1998; 87–107.*

32. Gibson CM, Murphy SA, Rizzo MJ, et al. Relationship between TIMI frame count and clinical outcomes after fibrinolytic administration. *Circulation 1999; 99:1945–1950.*

33. Gibson CM, Cannon CP, Murphy SA, et al. Relationship of TIMI myocardial perfusion grade to mortality after administration of fibrinolytic drugs. *Circulation 2000; 101:125–130.*

34. Tennant R, Wiggers CJ. The effect of coronary occlusion on myocardial contraction. *Am J Physiol 1935; 112:351–361.*

35. Reimer KA, Lowe JE, Rasmussen MM, Jennings RB. The wavefront phenomenon of ischemic cell death. 1: Myocardial infarct size vs. duration of coronary occlusion in dogs. *Circulation 1977; 56:786–794.*

36. Bergman SR, Lerch RA, Fox KAA, et al. Temporal dependence of beneficial effects of coronary fibrinolysis characterized by positron tomography. *Am J Med 1982; 73:573–581.*

37. Fibrinolytic Therapy Trialists' (FTT) Collaborative Group. Indications for fibrinolytic therapy in suspected acute myocardial infarction: collaborative overview of early mortality and major morbidity results from all randomised trials of more than 1000 patients. *Lancet 1994; 343: 311–322.*

38. LATE Study Group. Late Assessment of Thrombolytic Efficacy (LATE) study with alteplase 6–24 hours after onset of acute myocardial infarction. *Lancet 1993; 342:759–766.*

39. Rogers WJ, Bowlby LJ, Chandra NC, et al. Treatment of myocardial infarction in the United States (1990 to 1993): observations from the National Registry of Myocardial Infarction. *Circulation 1994; 90: 2103–2114.*

40. NHAAP Recommendations: Educational strategies to prevent pre-hospital delay in patients at high risk for acute myocardial infarction. *Washington, DC: U.S. Department of Health NIH Publication. 1997; 97–3787.*

41. Cannon CP, Gibson M, Lambrew CT, et al. Relationship of symptom-onset-to-ballon time and door-to-balloon time with mortality in patients undergoing angioplasty for acute myocardial infarction. *JAMA 2000; 283:2941–2947.*

42. International Joint Efficacy Comparison of Thrombolytic. Randomized, double-blinded comparison of reteplase double-bolus administration with streptokinase in acute myocardial infarction (INJECT): trial to investigate equivalence. *Lancet 1995; 346:329–336.*

43. Bode C, Smalling RW, Berg G, et al. Randomized comparison of coronary thrombolysis achieved with double-bolus reteplase (recombinant plasminogen activator) and front-loaded, accelerated alteplase (recombinant tissue plasminogen activator) in patients with acute myocardial infarction. *Circulation 1996; 4:891–898.*

44. The Global Use of Strategies to Open Occluded Coronary Arteries (GUSTO III) Investigators. A comparison of reteplase with alteplase for acute myocardial infarction. *N Engl J Med. 1997; 337:118–1123.*

45. Keyt BA, Paoni NF, Refino CJ, et al. A faster-acting and more potent form of tissue plasminogen activator. *Proc Natl Acad Sci USA 1994; 91:3670–3674.*

46. Cannon CP, Gibson CM, McCabe CH, et al. TNK-tissue plasminogen activator compared with front-loaded alteplase in acute myocardial infarction: results of the TIMI-10B trial. *Circulation 1998; 98:2805– 2814.*

47. The Assessment of the Safety and Efficacy of a New Thrombolytic (ASSENT-2) Investigator. Single-bolus tenecteplase compared with front-loaded alteplase in acute myocardial infarction: the ASSENT-2 double-blind randomized trial. *Lancet 1999; 354:715–722.*

48. Antman EM, Giogliano RP, Gibson CM, et al. Abciximab facilitates the rate and extent of fibrinolysis: Results of the Thrombolysis in Myocardial Infarction (TIMI) 14 trial. *Circulation 1999; 99:2720–2732.*

49. The GUSTO V Investigators. Reperfusion therapy for acute myocardial infarction with fibrinolytic therapy or combination reduced fibrinolytic therapy and platelet glycoprotein IIb/IIa inhibition: the GUSTO V randomised trial. *Lancet 2001; 357:1905–14.*

50. The Assessment of the Safety and Efficacy of a New Thrombolytic Regimen (ASSENT-3) Investigators. Efficacy and safety of tenecteplase in combination with enoxaparin, abciximab, or unfractionated heparin: the ASSENT-3 randomized trial in acute myocardial infarction. *Lancet 2001; 358:605–13.*

51. Ryan TJ, Antman EM, Brooks NH, et al. Update: ACC/AHA guidelines for the management of patients with acute myocardial infarction: a report of the American College of Cardiology/American Heart Association Task Force on Practice Guidelines (Committee on Management of Acute Myocardial Infarction). *J Am Coll Cardiol 1999; 34:890–911.*

52. Hartzler GO, Rutherford BD, McConahay DR, et al. Percutaneous transluminal coronary angioplasty with and without thrombolytic therapy for treatment of acute myocardial infarction. *Am Heart J 1983; 106:965–973.*

53. Grines CI, Browne KF, Maraco J, et al. A comparison of immediate angioplasty with fibrinolytic therapy for acute myocardial infarction: the primary angioplasty in myocardial infarction study group. *N Eng J Med 1993; 328:673–679.*

54. Hochman JS, Sleeper LA, Webb JG, et al. Early revascularization in acute myocardial infarction complicated by cardiogenic shock: SHOCK Investigators: Should we emergently revascularize occluded coronaries for cardiogenic shock. *N Eng J Med 1999; 341:625–634.*

55. Keeley EC, Boura JA, Grines CL. Primary angioplasty versus intravenous thrombolytic therapy for acute myocardial infarction: a quantitative review of 23 randomized trials. *Lancet 2003; 361:13–20.*

56. Canto JG, Every NR, Magid DJ, Rogers WJ, Malmgren JA, Frederick PD, French WJ, Tiefenbrunn AJ, Misra VK, Kiefe CI, Barron HV (for the National Registry of Myocardial Infarction 2 Investigators). The volume of primary angioplasty procedures and survival after acute myocardial infarction. *NEJM 2001; 342(21):1573–80.*

57. Magid DJ, Calonge BN, Runsfeld JS, Canto JG, Frederick PD, Every NR, Barron HV (for the National Registry of Myocardial Infarction 2 and 3 Investigators) Relation between hospital primary angioplasty volume and mortality for patients with acute MI treated with primary angioplasty vs. thrombolytic therapy. *JAMA 2000; 284:3131–3138 (NRMI 2 & 3).*

58. Dauerman HL, Sobel BE. Synergistic treatment of ST segment elevation myocardial infarction with pharmacoinvasive recanalization. *J. Am. Coll. Cardiol. 42:646–651, 2003.*

59. Ross AM, Coyne KA, Reiner JS et al. A randomized trial comparing primary angioplasty with a strategy of short-acting fibrinolysis and immediate planned rescue angioplasty in acute myocardial infarction: the PACT trial. *J Am Coll Cardiol. 1999; 34: 1954–1962.*

60. Barron HV, Bowlby LJ, Breen T, et al. Use of reperfusion therapy for acute myocardial infarction in the United States: data from the National Registry of Myocardial Infarction 2. *Circulation 1998; 97:1150–1156.*

3

The United Arab Emirates Experience: Treatment of Patients with Acute ST Elevation Myocardial Infarction with Thrombolytic Drugs

AZAN S. BINBREK and NAYAN S. RAO

Rashid Hospital
Dubai, U.A.E.

I. INTRODUCTION

In patients with acute ST segment elevation myocardial infarction (STEMI), early recanalization of the infarct-related artery (IRA) is crucial. In the past three decades, several randomized clinical trials have shown that thrombolysis redues morbidity and mortality (1–3). In the past decade, primary percutaneous coronary intervention (PCI) has been shown to be as effective as or more effective than thrombolysis in reducing the incidence of cardiac events after an index infarct. An ongoing debate swirls around which of these two treatment regimens is the preferred one. In this context, our experience in treating patients with STEMI virtually exclusively with pharmacological thrombolysis may be illuminating.

II. METHODS AND MATERIALS

From 1995 through 2002, we participated in four international randomized studies and one collaborative study with the University of Vermont in which pharmacological thrombolysis was employed with alteplase [tissue-type plasminogen activator (t-PA)] or tenecteplase [TNK–t-PA (TNK)]. In this chapter we summarize our experience with the cohorts of patients in all of these studies who were studied in the United Arab Emirates (UAE). The first of the studies was the Continuous Infusion versus Double Bolus of Alteplase (COBALT) study. The other three were Assessment of the Safety and Efficacy of a New Thrombolytic (ASSENT I, II, III) studies and a substudy in ASSENT II with the University of Vermont (4–8). The last study, a collaborative one with the University of Vermont, was the Enhanced Rapidity of RECanalization with Tenecteplase compared with Alteplase (ERRECTA) study, results of which have not yet been published. All of the patients participating in ERRECTA were patients in the UAE.

In the COBALT study, front-loaded infusion of alteplase was compared with use of a double bolus of alteplase. Results showed equivalence in the two groups with a slightly increased incidence of hemorrhage in the double bolus group (4). ASSENT I evaluated the safety of several doses of a then novel thrombolytic agent, TNK, given as a single bolus to patients with acute myocardial infarction. The overall safety profile of a single bolus of 30–50 mg TNK was found to be comparable to that of front-loaded t-PA observed in other large trials (5). ASSENT II was a double-blind randomized controlled trial designed to assess the efficacy and safety of TNK compared with t-PA. TNK and t-PA yielded equivalent results with respect to 30-day mortality. The ease of administration of TNK may facilitate more rapid treatment either before hospitalization or in the hospital (6). ASSENT III was a randomized open-label trial designed to compare the efficacy and safety of TNK plus enoxaparin or abciximab with that of TNK plus weight-adjusted unfractionated heparin in patients with acute myocardial infarction. The TNK plus enoxaparin or abciximab regimens studied in the UAE reduced the frequency of ischaemic complications of an acute myocardial infarction (7). We also conducted a substudy in ASSENT II to compare the relative rapidity of recanalization induced by t-PA and TNK assessed with enzymatic methods (8). The results showed very early recanalization (within 40 minutes after onset of administration of the thrombolytic agent) in 56% of patients who were given t-PA and 76% of patients who were given TNK.

We enrolled a total of 1030 patients in these studies in aggregate, all of whom were admitted within 6 hours after the onset of symptoms and signs of acute myocardial infarction. The patients were studied in three hospitals in the UAE. The inclusion criteria comprised an age of 18 years or greater; onset of symptoms within 6 hours before randomization; ST segment elevation of 0.1 mv in two or more electrocardiographic limb leads, 0.2 mv in two or more contiguous precordial electrocardiographic leads, or left bundle branch block; and chest pain persisting for 30 minutes and consistent with acute myocardial infarction. Exclusion criteria were severe hypertension (systolic blood pressure exceeding 180 mmHg or diastolic blood pressure exceeding 110 mmHg) on repeated measurements; use of a glycoprotein IIb/IIIa antagonist within the preceding 12 hours; major surgery, biopsy of a parenchymal organ, or a substantial trauma within the preceding 2 months; any major head trauma or other trauma occurring after onset of symptoms of the index myocardial infarction; any history of stroke, transient ischemic attacks, or dementia; any nonstructural damage to the central nervous system; current treatment with oral anticoagulants resulting in international normalized ratio of more than 1.3; sustained (>10 min) cardiopulmonary resuscitation in the preceding 2 weeks; pregnancy; lactation or parturition in the past 30 days with women of childbearing potential having had a negative pregnancy test; any participation in another investigational drug or device study within the previous 30 days; previous participation in the present study; any disorder that the investigator judged would place the patient at increased risk; and inability to follow the protocol or to comply with requirements for follow-up. The protocols were approved by institutional review boards at all institutions participating in the study and by the regulatory authorities of the UAE. Following acquisition of written informed consent, the patients were enrolled.

Many in the overall population of the UAE are young, with only 2% above the age of 50 years and 60% within the 30–50 years of age group. The population is predominantly male (70%) (9). This

Table 3.1   Baseline Characteristics of Patients in UAE Centers

Characteristics	
n	1030
Female (%)	2.5
Mean age (y)	47.2 ± 8.6
>75 years old (%)	0.8
Mean weight (kg)	71.2 ± 12.3
Mean BMI (kg/m2)	25.7 ± 3.9
Smoking status	
Nonsmokers (%)	47.9
Current smokers (%)	52.1
Prior MI (%)	9.3
Previous Hx. hypertension (%)	22.3
Previous Hx. diabetes (%)	29
Median time from symptoms onset to treatment (h)	3.25[a]

[a] ASSENT I patients were excluded from this calculation because of differences in exclusion criteria (time from symptoms onset to treatment >12 h) compared with other UAE patients and studies.

demographic imbalance is attributable to a large expatriate population comprising predominantly single and young males from the Indian subcontinent. Throughout the UAE, patients with chest pain proceed directly to hospital emergency departments. Distances required for transport to hospital are short.

Following acquisition of written informed consent, 1030 patients were studied, 97.5% of whom were male. The mean age was 47.2 years; 29% of the patients had overt diabetes, 52.1% were current smokers, 22.3% had previously diagnosed hypertension (BP > 140/80 mmHg), mean BMI was 25.7 (±3.9), and 9.3% had sustained a previous myocardial infarction. All were admitted within 6 hours following the onset of chest pain, most very early (mean = 195 minutes) (Tables 3.1–3.6).

The incidences of adverse outcomes of 30-day mortality, reinfarction, stroke, and major bleeding were extremely low compared with global experience. The 30-day mortality was 3.1%; less than 1% of the patients sustained a stroke; only 0.3% had a hemorrhagic stroke; 0.4% had an ischemic stroke; 0.1% had an unclassified stroke; and only 0.3% had cardiogenic shock (Table 3.7). There was no incidence of major bleeding requiring transfusion or laparotomy. In the ERRECTA study,

Table 3.2   Baseline Characteristics of UAE Patients in COBALT

Variable	
n	204
Female (%)	3.9
Mean age (y)	46.8 ± 8.6
>75 years old (%)	0.5
Mean weight (kg)	72 ± 12.4
Mean BMI (kg/m²)	25.8 ± 3.7
Smoking status	
Nonsmokers (%)	46.6
Current smokers (%)	53.4
Prior MI (%)	NA
Previous Hx. hypertension (%)	NA
Previous Hx. diabetes (%)	NA
Median time from symptoms onset to treatment (h)	3.5[a]

[a] Median time from symptom onset to treatment for ASSENT I patients was not considered (time from symptoms onset to treatment > 12 h.)

Table 3.3   Baseline Characteristics of UAE Patients in ASSENT I

Characteristics	
n	154
Female (%)	3.3
Mean age (y)	46.4 ± 8.3
>75 years old (%)	0
Mean (SD) weight (kg)	71.2 ± 13.6
Mean BMI (kg/m²)	25.6 ± 8.3
Smoking status	
Nonsmokers (%)	48.8
Current smokers (%)	55.2
Prior MI (%)	9.1
Previous Hx. hypertension (%)	20.8
Previous Hx. diabetes (%)	24.2

we found that TNK induced recanalization even more rapidly than did t-PA (Tables 3.7–3.12). Overall 30-day mortality was significantly lower ($p = 0.03$) in those patients who were treated within 3 hours or less of the onset of symptoms (2.1%) compared with that in those

Table 3.4 Baseline Characteristics of UAE Patients in ASSENT II

Characteristics	
n	218
Female (%)	2.3
Mean (SD) age (y)	47.4 ± 8.8
>75 years old (%)	0.9
Mean (SD) weight (kg)	71 ± 11.4
Mean (SD) BMI (kg/m^2)	25.5 ± 3.6
Smoking Status	
Nonsmokers (%)	40.2
Current smokers (%)	59.8
Prior MI (%)	14.2
Previous Hx. hypertension (%)	24.8
Previous Hx. diabetes (%)	26.1
Median time from symptoms onset to treatment (h)	3.5

Table 3.5 Baseline Characteristics of UAE Patients in ASSENT III

Characteristics	
n	184
Female (%)	2.2
Mean age (y)	48 ± 8.6
>75 years old (%)	0.54
Mean weight (kg)	71.2 ± 12.4
Mean BMI (kg/m^2)	25.5 ± 3.8
Smoking status	
Nonsmokers (%)	44
Current smokers (%)	56
Prior MI (%)	7.1
Previous Hx. hypertension (%)	22.3
Previous Hx. diabetes (%)	29.3
Median time from symptoms onset to treatment (h)	3.3

patients treated between 3 and 6 hours after the onset of symptoms (3.6%) (Table 3.13).

III. DISCUSSION

Our results in 1030 patients with STEMI treated in our own center with either t-PA or TNK in the five clinical trials between 1995 and 2002

Table 3.6   Baseline Characteristics of ERRECTA Participants

Characteristics	
n	270
Female (%)	1.4
Mean (SD) age (y)	48
[95% CI]	
>75 years old (%)	NA
Mean weight (kg)	70.8 ± 12.2
Mean BMI (kg/m²)	25.9 ± 3.9
Smoking status	
Nonsmokers (%)	45.2
Current smokers (%)	54.8
Prior MI (%)	7.0
Previous Hx. hypertension (%)	21.0
Previous Hx. diabetes (%)	34
Mean time from symptoms onset to treatment (h)	3

Table 3.7   Outcomes for All UAE Patients

Outcomes	n	%
Number of participants	1030	
Total death within 30 days	32	3.1
Reinfarction	36	3.5
Moderate bleeding	9	0.9
Stroke	8	0.8
Hemorrhagic	3	0.3
Ischemic	4	0.4
Unclassified	1	0.1
Cardiogenic shock	3	0.3

show a strikingly low morbidity and mortality following treatment with both agents. Our patients were relatively young compared with those in many trials. This would favor a low mortality. Nevertheless, in the population studied many risk factors were prevalent including hypertension, obesity, smoking, previous infarction, and diabetes (a prevalence twice that typical in western Europe and North America). In the UAE the prevalence of diabetes is 18.9% (10).

Table 3.8 Outcomes for UAE
Patients in Cobalt

Outcomes	n	%
Number of participants	204	
Total death	4	1.7
Reinfarction	5	2.5
Moderate bleeding	2	1.0
Stroke	0	0
Hemorrhagic	0	0
Ischemic	0	0
Unclassified	0	0
Cardiogenic shock	1	0.5

Table 3.9 Outcomes for UAE
Patients in ASSENT I

Outcomes	n	%
Number of participants	154	
Total death	2	1.3
Reinfarction	8	5.2
Moderate bleeding	3	1.9
Stroke	0	0
Hemorrhagic	0	0
Ischemic	0	0
Unclassified	0	0
Cardiogenic shock	0	0

Table 3.10 Outcomes for UAE
Patients in ASSENT II

Outcomes	n	%
Number of participants	218	
Total death	7	3.2
Reinfarction	7	3.2
Moderate bleeding	1	0.5
Stroke	0	0
Hemorrhagic	0	0
Ischemic	0	0
Unclassified	0	0
Cardiogenic shock	1	0.5

Table 3.11 Outcomes for UAE
Patients in ASSENT III

Outcomes	n	%
Number of participants	184	
Total death	12	6.5
Reinfarction	0	0
Moderate bleeding	0	0
Stroke	6	3.3
Hemorrhagic	2	1.1
Ischemic	3	1.6
Unclassified	1	0.5
Cardiogenic shock	0	0.0

Our patient population was predominantly male, consistent with
the demography of the UAE and the protection conferred in premeno-
pausal women from accelerated coronary artery disease as well as the
age distribution of the population. Thus, the number of women studied
was very low. Several studies have shown that when thrombolysis is
initiated less than 3 hours after the onset of chest pain, mortality is
remarkably low (11,12). Most of our patients were treated early. The
mean time from onset of chest pain to treatment was 3.25 hours. This
would, to some extent, account for the low mortality.

Table 3.12 Outcomes for Patients in ERRECTA

Outcomes	n	%
Number of participants	270	
Total death	7	2.6
Reinfarction	8	3.0
Moderate bleeding	1	0.4
Stroke	2	0.7
Hemorrhagic	1	0.4
Ischemic	1	0.4
Unclassified	0	0
Cardiogenic shock	1	0.4

Table 3.13 Overall 30-Day Mortality with Respect to Interval between Onset of Symptoms and Treatment

Time symptom onset to Rx (h)	Overall n	Mortality n (%)
0 to <3	421	9 (2.1)
3 to <6	552	20 (3.6)

Student t-test p-value = 0.0301.

In the UAE, as well as many countries in western Europe and North America, primary PCI for treatment of patients with STEMI was and still is not readily available in many hospitals. We believe the case for performing primary PCI in most such patients is not yet compelling. The impact of time to treatment on mortality after prehospital thrombolysis or primary angioplasty (CAPTIM study) has shown that prehospital thrombolysis may be preferable to primary PCI for patients treated within the first 2 hours after onset of symptoms. Conversely, the DANish Multi-Center Randomized Study on Fibrinolytic Therapy versus Acute Myocardial Infarction (DANAMI-2) report showed a reduction in cardiac events in patients treated with primary angioplasty compared with those treated with fibrinolytic agents for STEMI (13,14). The critics of that study have pointed out that the trial included only 37% of the population with STEMI and excluded patients with higher intervention-related mortality risks such as diabetes. All patients deemed to be a high risk during ambulance transport were excluded.

The clinical benefit of PCI demonstrated in randomized trials has not been replicated consistently in clinical practice. This may reflect differences in operator skills and experience and excessive delay in treatment in clinical practice (15).

We believe that pharmacoinvasive therapy in patients with STEMI is likely to emerge as the standard of care (16). It seems reasonable that those patients who present to hospital within 3 hours after the onset of chest pain should be offered treatment with a thrombolytic agent and that primary PCI should be reserved for those admitted relatively late (4 hours or more after onset of symptoms of STEMI), those with contraindications for thrombolysis, patients at high risk for death such as those above 70 years of age, patients in cardiogenic shock, and those with continuation of chest pain with persistent ST elevation or diabetes (17). Ongoing trials such as ASSENT IV/PCI may shed more light on the optimal way to proceed. In the interim, we should educate the public and emphasize the urgency of reaching the hospital as rapidly as possible. In our opinion, we should motivate triage staffs, ER physicians, and cardiologists to initiate treatment with thrombolytic agents as promptly as possible.

REFERENCES

1. TIMI Study Group. The Thrombolysis in Myocardial Infarction (TIMI) Trial. Phase I findings, N Engl J Med 1985; 312:932-936.

2. Gruppo Italiano per lo Studio della Streptochhinasi nell'Infarto Miocardico (GISSI). Effectiveness of intravenous thrombolytic treatment in acute myocardial infarction. Lancet 1986; 1:397-402.

3. Berger PB, Ellis SG, Holmes DR Jr, Granger CB, Criger DA, Betriu A, Topol EJ, Califf RM. Relationship between delay in performing direct coronary angioplasty and early clinical outcome in patients with acute myocardial infarction: results from the Global Use of Strategies to Open Occluded Arteries in Acute Coronary Syndrome (GUSTO-IIb) Trial. Circulation 1999; 100:14-20.

4. The Continuous Infusion versus Double-Bolus Administration of Alteplase (COBALT) Investigators. A comparison of continuous infusion of alteplase with double bolus administration for acute myocardial infarction. N Engl J Med 1997; 337:1127-1130.

5. Van de Werf F, Cannon C P, Luyten A, Houbracken K, McCabe CH, Be S, Bluhmki E, Srelin H, Wang-Clow F, Fox NL, Braunwald E. Safety assessment of single-bolus administration of TNK tissue-plasminogen activator in acute myocardial infarction: The ASSENT-I Trial. Am Heart J 1999; 137:786-791.

6. Assessment of the Safety and Efficacy of a New Thrombolytic (ASSENT-II) Investigators. Single-bolus tenecteplase compared with front-loaded alteplase in acute myocardial infarction: The ASSENT-II double blind randomized trial. Lancet 1999; 354:716-722.

7. Assessment of the Safety and Efficacy of a New Thrombolytic Regimen (ASSENT-III) Investigators. Efficacy and safety of tenecteplase in combination with enoxaparin, abciximab, or unfractionated heparin: The ASSENT-III randomized trial in acute myocardial infarction. Lancet 2001; 358:9282, 605-613.

8. Binbrek A, Rao N, Absher PM, Van de Werf F, Sobel BE. The relative rapidity of recanalization induced by recombinant tissue-type plasminogen activator (rt-PA) and TNK-tPA assessed with enzymatic methods. Coron Artery Dis 2000; 11:429-435.

9. Statistical Yearbook 2001. Dubai, United Arab Emirates, 2001.

10. Diabetes (Ministry of Health, unpublished date: Incidence of Diabetes in UAE, 2001).

11. Steg PG, Bonnefoy E, Chabaud S, Lapostolle F, Dubien PY, Cristofini P, Leizorovicz A, Touboul P. Impact of time to treatment on mortality after prehospital fibrinolysis or primary angioplasty. Data from the CAPTIM randomized clinical trial. Circulation 2003; 108:2851-2856.

12. Boersma E, Maas AC, Deckers JW, Simoons, ML. Early thrombolytic treatment in acute myocardial infarction: reappraisal of the golden hour. Lancet 1996; 348:771-775.

13. Andersen HR, Nielsen TT, Vesterlund T, Grande P, Abildgaard U, Thayssen P, Pedersen F, Mortensen LS, for the DANAMI-2 Investigators.

Danish multicenter randomized study on fibrinolytic therapy versus acute coronary angioplasty in acute myocardial infarction: rationale and design of the DANish trial in Acute Myocardial Infarction-2 (DAN-AMI-2). Am Heart J 2003; 146:234-241.

14. Widimsky P, Groch L, Zelizko M, Aschermann M, Bednar F, Suryaprai H. Multicentre randomized trial comparing transport to primary angioplasty versus immediate thrombolysis versus combined strategy for patients with acute myocardial infarction presenting to a community hospital without a catheterization laboratory. The PRAGUE study. Eur Heart J 2000; 21:823-831.

15. Welsh RC, Ornato J, Armstrong PW. Prehospital management of acute ST elevation myocardial infarction: a time for reappraisal in North America. Am Heart J 2003; 145:1-8.

16. Dauerman HL, Sobel BE. Synergistic treatment of ST segment elevation myocardial infarction with pharmacoinvasive recanalization. J Am Coll Cardiol 2003; 42:646-651.

17. Weaver WD. All hospitals are not equal for treatment of patients with acute myocardial infarction. Circulation 2003; 108:1768-1771.

4

Development, Impact, and Limitations of Primary Percutaneous Coronary Intervention for the Treatment of ST Elevation Myocardial Infarction

SIMON R. DIXON and
WILLIAM W. O'NEILL

William Beaumont Hospital,
Royal Oak, Michigan, U.S.A.

I. INTRODUCTION

In light of contemporary data, it is remarkable to consider that balloon angioplasty was first performed for acute myocardial infarction just 20 years ago. At that time angioplasty was still very much in its infancy for the treatment of coronary artery disease. It is perhaps not surprising, therefore, that initial attempts to use angioplasty in evolving myocardial infarction were met with widespread criticism. In fact, few other therapies in medicine have generated as much debate and controversy as primary angioplasty. Since those early days, however, extraordinary advances have been made in the development of mechanical reperfusion for myocardial infarction. Many of these major milestones can be attributed to a small but highly dedicated group of investigators in this field. On the basis of their pioneering work, catheter-based reperfusion has now emerged as the preferred reperfusion strategy for myocardial infarction. This chapter will review the key steps in the evolution of mechanical reperfusion as well as discuss the impact and limitations of primary percutaneous coronary intervention (PCI) in the current era.

II. THE EVOLUTION OF MECHANICAL REPERFUSION

A. Historical Background

Until the late 1970s, efforts to limit infarct size had focused almost exclusively on therapies designed to reduce cardiac afterload or myocardial metabolism. At that time angiographic studies in humans provided the first evidence that most cases of acute transmural myocardial infarction were indeed due to total coronary occlusion (1). Subsequently Rentrop and colleagues demonstrated that the infarct artery could be recanalized by intracoronary infusion of streptokinase (2). Together, these findings led to a major shift in research for myocardial infarction, thus ushering in the modern era of reperfusion. Within a short time, prospective randomized trials had confirmed the effectiveness of intracoronary fibrinolytic therapy to establish coronary patency as well as improve survival in patients with acute myocardial infarction (3,4).

B. The Dawn of Mechanical Reperfusion

The first cases of mechanical reperfusion were performed in 1978, using a conventional guidewire to recanalize the infarct vessel (5,6). Shortly thereafter, balloon angioplasty emerged as a new treatment modality for obstructive coronary disease. Several groups promptly recognized the potential role for angioplasty to mechanically restore flow in the culprit vessel during evolving myocardial infarction. In the early 1980s, a number of observational studies confirmed the feasibility of balloon angioplasty in this setting, with or without prior thrombolytic therapy (7,8). The necessity of antecedent thrombolysis soon came into question and led to a prospective, randomized trial comparing the merits

Table 4.1 Randomized Trials of Immediate PTCA after Intravenous Thrombolytic Therapy

	TAMI-1 (n = 386)		TIMI-IIA (n = 389)		ECSG (n = 367)	
PTCA strategy	Immediate	Day 7	Immediate	18–24 h	Immediate	None
Transfusion (%)	NR	NR	20	7	10	4
Emergency CABG (%)	7	2	4	2	NR	NR
LV ejection fraction (%)	53	56	50	49	51	51
Mortality (%)	4	1	7	5	7	3

NR = Not reported.

of each therapeutic strategy. The Ann Arbor group demonstrated that coronary angioplasty resulted in less recurrent ischemia and greater recovery of ventricular function than intracoronary streptokinase (9). However, coronary angioplasty was still in its infancy, and a number of logistic constraints, including lack of trained operators and catheterization facilities, hindered widespread adoption of this technique.

C. The Strep-and-Stretch Approach

With completion of the GISSI and ISIS-2 trials in the mid-1980s, intravenous fibrinolysis was rapidly adopted as the first-line reperfusion strategy for myocardial infarction (10,11). However, the early studies of intracoronary thrombolysis had shown that most patients still had a severe residual stenosis after successful thrombolysis (12). Many investigators remained concerned about the risk of reocclusion of the infarct vessel and thought that angioplasty should be performed routinely after thrombolysis even in asymptomatic patients. This became known as the strep-and-stretch approach.

Three prospective, randomized trials were performed in the late 1980s to determine if routine angioplasty would reduce the incidence of reocclusion or reinfarction, or augment recovery of ventricular function after thrombolysis (13–15). The results of these trials were surprising and disappointing (Table 4.1). Patients assigned to routine angioplasty had a higher incidence of adverse events including a higher transfusion rate and need for emergency bypass surgery as well as a trend toward increased mortality (16). On the basis of these data, the strategy of routine immediate angioplasty after thrombolytic therapy was abandoned following these trials. However, there were a number of important limitations with these studies, which preclude extrapolation of these data to the present mechanical reperfusion era. Notably, some of these studies failed to give preprocedural aspirin or administer adequate doses of heparin, both of which are known to increase the risk of abrupt vessel closure. In addition, there was a failure to monitor ACTs, and in some cases treatment of noncritical coronary stenoses was also permitted. Since that time there have been extraordinary advances in the interventional therapy of myocardial infarction. These changes have dramatically improved the safety and long-term outcome of these procedures.

D. The Emergence of Primary PTCA

The trials of angioplasty performed immediately after thrombolysis had a profound impact on the further development of mechanical reperfusion. Based on these findings, there was widespread opinion that post-thrombolytic angioplasty was potentially harmful and should be discouraged as a reperfusion strategy. At the same time there was tremendous enthusiasm for newer, more effective second-generation fibrinolytic agents (17). As a result, the paths of mechanical and pharmacological reperfusion diverged, and within a short time, both were viewed as competing, rather than complimentary, strategies. Although momentum slowed somewhat, many centers firmly believed that primary PCI had been inadequately tested as a reperfusion strategy. This prompted the need for well-designed prospective randomized trials to define the efficacy of primary PCI compared with intravenous fibrinolysis.

E. The Reperfusion Wars

In the early 1990s 10 randomized trials were performed comparing primary angioplasty to thrombolytic therapy (18–27). The largest of these were the PAMI-1, Zwolle, and Gusto-IIb trials (18,23,27). Although there was marked heterogeneity between these trials in terms of study design and thrombolytic agent used, most of these studies demonstrated superior clinical outcomes with mechanical reperfusion.

The PAMI-1 trial randomized 395 patients to angioplasty or t-PA within 12 hours of the onset of myocardial infarction (23). Compared to the t-PA group, patients assigned to primary angioplasty had a significantly lower incidence of in-hospital death or nonfatal reinfarction (5.1% vs. 12.0%; $p = 0.02$), less recurrent ischemia (10.3% vs. 28.0%; $p < 0.001$), and a lower risk of intracranial hemorrhage (0 vs. 2.0%; $p = 0.05$). Similar results were also seen in the larger GUSTO-IIb trial, which randomized 1138 patients to angioplasty or accelerated t-PA (27). In this study, primary angioplasty was associated with a 33% reduction in the primary endpoint of death, reinfarction, or disabling stroke at 30 days (13.7% vs. 9.6%; $p = 0.03$). However, the late results were less impressive. In contrast to the PAMI-1 and Zwolle trials, no significant clinical advantage was seen with angioplasty at 6 months. These discordant results may have been related to the fact that angioplasty was performed less often in patients randomized to the procedure in GUSTO-IIb than PAMI-1 and was also associated with a lower rate of final TIMI 3 flow in the infarct vessel.

Despite the results of the PAMI and Zwolle trials, great controversy persisted regarding the relative benefit of catheter-based reperfusion versus fibrinolytic therapy for acute myocardial infarction. Primary PTCA was regarded as a reasonable alternative to fibrinolytic therapy but was not widely employed due to logistical problems and relative paucity of data to support its clinical benefit. It took a further decade of clinical research to settle this controversy.

F. Stent Implantation: The Next Big Advance

The main factor limiting the efficacy of primary angioplasty is restenosis and reocclusion of the infarct-related artery. Adjunctive stenting emerged as a promising means of improving early and late outcomes after mechanical reperfusion. However, stenting was initially avoided in acute myocardial infarction because of concern about the risk of stent thrombosis. It was not until the importance of optimal stent deployment and effective platelet inhibition was recognized that primary stenting became feasible. Initial pilot studies confirmed the safety of stenting in myocardial infarction and paved the way for prospective, randomized trials.

Seven randomized studies comparing primary stenting to angioplasty in acute myocardial infarction have been reported (28–34). It is important to note that these trials differ markedly with respect to sample size, stent design, crossover rates, and use of adjunctive glycoprotein receptor antagonists (Table 4.2). In general, most of these studies have demonstrated superior clinical results with stenting compared to balloon angioplasty alone, primarily due to a reduction in angiographic restenosis and reocclusion of the infarct vessel (Table 4.3).

In the Stent-PAMI trial, 900 patients with infarct vessels suitable for stenting were randomized to angioplasty alone or angioplasty with stent implantation (32). Stenting resulted in a larger minimal lumen diameter, less residual stenosis, and fewer dissections than angioplasty alone. At 6 months, stenting was associated with a lower incidence of the combined endpoint of death, reinfarction, disabling stroke, or target vessel revascularization (12.6% vs. 20.1%; $p < 0.01$). This was primarily due to a lower rate of target vessel revascularization in the stent group (7.7% vs. 17.0%; $p < 0.001$). Furthermore, stenting was associated with a lower incidence of restenosis compared to angioplasty alone (20.3% vs. 33.5%; $p < 0.001$).

Despite these encouraging data, enthusiasm for routine stent implantation was tempered by the fact that stenting was associated with a lower rate of final TIMI 3 flow (89% vs. 93%; $p = 0.006$) and a higher 12-month mortality than balloon angioplasty alone (5.8% vs. 3.1%; $p = 0.07$) (Figs. 4.1 and 4.2). Concern was raised that stenting might increase the risk of distal embolization as a result of the bulky stent-delivery system or high-pressure postdilatation. For these reasons it was recommended that stenting be reserved for patients with a suboptimal angiographic result or dissection following balloon angioplasty.

Fortunately, these concerns were alleviated after the results of the larger CADILLAC trial were reported (34). In contrast to previous trials, this was the only study to use a second-generation stent design and include adjunctive therapy with a glycoprotein receptor antagonist. In this trial 2082 patients with an infarct artery stenosis of >70% and vessel diameter of 2.5–3.75 mm were randomized to one of four treatment arms: stenting (with or without abciximab) or angioplasty (with or without abciximab). Angiographic exclusion criteria included unprotected left main disease (>60% stenosis), culprit vessel in a saphenous

Table 4.2 Randomized Trials of Stenting Compared to Angioplasty in Acute Myocardial Infarction: Study Design

Trial (Ref.)	Year	n	Patient population	Duration of symptoms	Design	Stent type	Randomization	Bailout stent n (%)
GRAMI (28)	1998	104	ST↑ <75 y CS included	<24 h	Multicenter	GR II	After culprit lesion crossed with guidewire	13 (25)
FRESCO (29)	1998	150	ST↑ CS included	<6 h 6–12 h if ongoing ischemia	Single center	GR-II, PS, microstent	After optimal PTCA result	—
Zwolle (30)	1998	227	ST↑	<6 h 6–12 h if ongoing ischemia	Single center	PS	After guidewire or balloon induced reperfusion	15 (13)
PASTA (31)	1999	136	ST↑	<12 h	Multicenter	PS	After diagnostic angiography	7 (10)
Stent-PAMI (32)	1999	900	ST↑	<12 h	Multicenter	Heparin-coated PS	After reperfusion (spontaneous or PTCA)	15%
STENTIM (33)	2000	211	ST↑	<12 h	Multicenter	Wiktor	After diagnostic angiography	36.4%
CADILLAC (34)	2002	2082	ST↑	<12 h	Multicenter	MultiLink and MultiLink Duet	After diagnostic angiography	NR

CS = Cardiogenic shock; GR II= Gianturco-Roubin II stent; PS = Palmaz-Schatz stent.

Table 4.3   Randomized Trials of Stenting Compared to Angioplasty in Acute Myocardial Infarction: 6-Month Results

Trial (Ref.)	Year	Target vessel revascularization			Death, MI, and TVR		
		PTCA	Stent	*p*-value	PTCA	Stent	*p*-value
GRAMI[a] (28)	1998	7.0	0	NS	19.2	3.8	0.03
FRESCO (29)	1998	25.0	7.0	0.002	28.0	9.0	0.003
Zwolle (30)	1998	17.0	4.0	0.0016	20.0	5.4	0.001
PASTA[b] (31)	1999	13.0	6.0	NS	46.0	21.0	<0.001
Stent-PAMI[c] (32)	1999	17.0	7.7	<0.001	20.1	12.6	0.01
STENTIM (33)	2000	26.4	16.8	NS	32.9	24.8	NS
CADILLAC Abciximab + (34)	2002	13.8	5.2	<0.001	16.5	10.2	<0.001
CADILLAC Abciximab – (34)	2002	15.7	8.3		20.0	11.5	

TVR = Ischemia-driven target vessel revascularization.
[a] GRAMI = In-hospital outcomes.
[b] Target lesion revascularization.
[c] Composite endpoint includes disabling stroke.

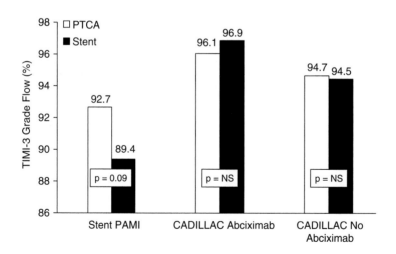

Figure 4.1   Rate of TIMI 3 flow in the infarct-related artery after primary angioplasty or stent implantation in the Stent-PAMI (32) and CADILLAC (34) trials.

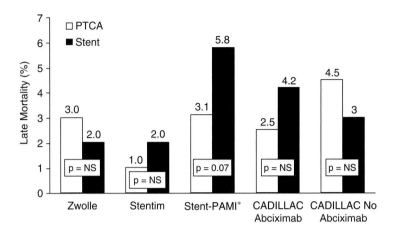

Figure 4.2 Late mortality in randomized trials of angioplasty or stenting for acute myocardial infarction (6-month follow-up except for Stent-PAMI = 1-year follow-up). (From Refs. 30,32–34.)

vein or internal mammary graft, presence of a major side branch, or need for multivessel PCI during the acute phase. At 6 months there was a significant improvement in event-free survival with MultiLink stent implantation compared to angioplasty with bailout stenting (primary endpoint of MACE 10.9% vs. 19.3%; $p = 0.001$) (Fig. 4.3). This benefit was primarily due to a reduction in the incidence of target vessel revascularization. Importantly, stenting was not associated with a reduction in TIMI 3 flow as seen in the Stent-PAMI trial, and no difference in late mortality was observed between any of the treatment arms. On the basis of these results, routine primary stenting is recommended in patients undergoing mechanical reperfusion for acute myocardial infarction. Balloon angioplasty alone remains an excellent strategy when either an optimal angiographic result can be achieved or the patient has coronary anatomy that is unfavorable for stent implantation.

G. Adjunctive Pharmacotherapy

The introduction of glycoprotein IIb/IIIa receptor antagonists in the mid-1990s was an important advance in adjunctive pharmacological therapy for mechanical reperfusion. Preliminary data were reported

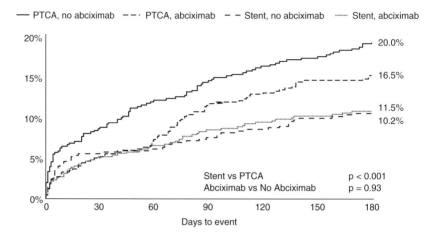

Figure 4.3 Incidence of major adverse cardiac events (death, myocardial infarction, disabling stroke, or ischemia-driven target vessel revascularization) at 6 months in the CADILLAC trial (34).

from a small subset of patients with acute myocardial infarction in the EPIC trial and suggested that treatment with abciximab had a favorable clinical benefit (35,36). Since then, five randomized trials have evaluated the efficacy of abciximab during either primary balloon angioplasty or primary stenting for acute myocardial infarction (Table 4.4) (37–41). Overall, these data suggest that abciximab has a salutary effect on early and late clinical outcomes. However, results of these trials have been rather discordant, and this has led to intense controversy regarding the indication for abciximab, particularly during stent implantation. Notably, there are several important differences between these trials with respect to study design and inclusion criteria that may account for some of the variation in trial results. Debate has centered mainly on the question of whether abciximab should be administered *routinely* during mechanical reperfusion (42). Three trials (ACE, ADMIRAL, and ISAR-2) have demonstrated a significant benefit with abciximab therapy during stent implantation (38–40). The greatest benefit was observed in the ADMIRAL trial, in which abciximab was given *early* before cardiac catheterization. In addition, the ADMIRAL trial

Table 4.4 Randomized Trials of Abciximab with Primary PTCA or Stenting for Acute Myocardial Infarction: Composite Clinical Endpoint at 30 Days

Study (Ref.)	Year	Study design	n	Abciximab (%)	Placebo (%)	p-value
PTCA						
RAPPORT (37)	1998	AMI <12 h, nonshock	483	13.3	16.1	0.32
CADILLAC (PTCA) (34)	2002	AMI <12 h, nonshock	1046	4.8	8.3	0.02
Stent						
ADMIRAL (38)	2000	AMI <12 h, CS included	300	6.0	14.6	0.01
ISAR-2 (39)	2000	AMI <48 h, CS included	401	5.0	10.5	0.04
CADILLAC (Stent) (34)	2002	AMI <12 h, nonshock	1036	4.4	5.7	NS
ACE (40)	2003	AMI <24 h, CS included	400	4.5	10.5	0.02

CS = Cardiogenic shock.

demonstrated a higher left ventricular ejection fraction in abciximab-treated patients. The largest trial, CADILLAC, also showed an improvement in the composite endpoint of death, reinfarction, and target vessel revascularization at 30 days, but most of this benefit was seen in patients treated with balloon angioplasty alone. In contrast to the other studies, abciximab did not confer any benefit on major adverse cardiac events in stented patients. Moreover, there was no benefit of abciximab on convalescent ventricular function at 7 months. Abciximab was associated with a reduction in the incidence of subacute thrombosis in stented patients (0.0% vs. 1.0%; $p = 0.03$). Fewer studies are available with other glycoprotein IIb/IIIa inhibitors.

III. OVERVIEW OF RANDOMIZED TRIALS OF ANGIOPLASTY AND THROMBOLYSIS

In 2003 Keeley and Grines performed a careful meta-analysis of 23 randomized trials comparing angioplasty and thrombolytic therapy for

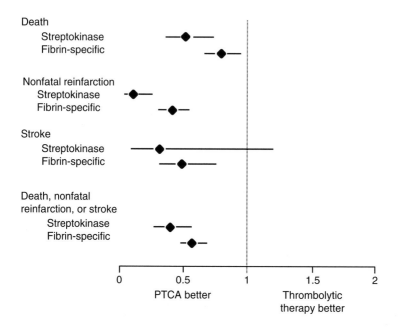

Figure 4.4 Short-term clinical outcomes in individuals treated with PTCA or thrombolytic therapy, according to type of thrombolytic agent used. Odds ratios and 95% CI are shown. (From Ref. 43.)

acute myocardial infarction (43). In this overview, primary PCI was associated with a lower short-term mortality (5% vs. 7%; $p = 0.0002$), lower incidence of nonfatal reinfarction (3% vs. 7%; $p < 0.0001$), and lower incidence of stroke (1% vs. 2%; $p = 0.0004$) (Fig. 4.4). Compared with thrombolysis, the estimated survival benefit with PCI was 21 lives saved per 1000 patients treated. The benefit of angioplasty was independent of the type of thrombolytic agent used (streptokinase or fibrin-specific agents). Angioplasty was associated with a dramatically lower incidence of intracranial hemorrhage than thrombolysis (0.05% vs. 1.1%; $p < 0.0001$), but the overall risk of major bleeding (mostly related to access site bleeding) was higher with PCI (7% vs. 5%; $p = 0.032$). A lower risk of bleeding was noted in the 13 most recent trials, attributable to lower doses of intravenous heparin, smaller sheath sizes, and improved operator technique. The relative treatment effect appears to be similar across all subgroups of patients (44).

A. Primary PCI in Thrombolytic Ineligible Patients

Observational studies have demonstrated that patients with contraindications to thrombolytic therapy have a particularly high mortality (45,46). Recent data from the National Registry of Myocardial Infarction (NRMI) database indicate that the mortality benefit of mechanical revascularization also extends to this high-risk group (47). In this propensity analysis, patients who were selected to receive immediate revascularization had a 46% relative reduction in the risk of hospital mortality compared to patients who did not undergo revascularization (10.9% vs. 20.1%; OR 0.48, 95% CI 0.43–0.55). More importantly, the study also provided insight into the alarmingly low utilization of mechanical reperfusion in thrombolytic ineligible patients. Of the 19,917 patients in the study, only 4707 (24%) underwent revascularization. Overall, these findings strongly support routine adoption of mechanical reperfusion for thrombolytic ineligible patients as well as the need to improve access to centers with invasive facilities.

B. High-Risk Patient Groups

Patients with high-risk clinical features, including anterior infarction, advanced age, prior bypass surgery, and cardiogenic shock, derive the greatest absolute benefit from mechanical reperfusion therapy (48–52). Elderly patients in particular, who have a much higher rate of stroke and intracranial bleeding with thrombolytic therapy, appear to have a substantial mortality benefit with primary PCI (53). Patients with prior coronary artery bypass surgery should also be considered for mechanical recanalization (54–58). Reperfusion rates with thrombolytic therapy are significantly lower in acute saphenous vein graft occlusion than in native vessels due, in part, to the larger thrombotic burden in vein grafts. On the other hand, mechanical reperfusion achieves TIMI 3 flow in approximately 70% of saphenous vein graft culprits. Clinical outcomes may be further improved by adjunctive use of thrombectomy or distal protection devices.

Catheter-based reperfusion is the preferred treatment strategy for patients with cardiogenic shock complicating acute myocardial infarction. In this setting, hypotension markedly reduces the efficacy of thrombolytic therapy to restore epicardial flow (59). The GISSI-1 trial is the only placebo-controlled study of thrombolytic therapy that included patients with cardiogenic shock (10). In this 280-patient subgroup, there was no difference in 30-day mortality for patients treated with streptokinase or placebo (70.1% vs. 69.9%). More recently, the 302-patient randomized SHOCK trial has provided compelling evidence for invasive therapy versus medical stabilization in cardiogenic shock (60). At 6 months there was a significantly lower mortality in the patients treated with early revascularization (50% vs. 63%; $p = 0.027$), especially in those treated within 6 hours of symptom onset, patients <75 years of age, and patients with prior myocardial infarction. However, mortality remains extremely high in this group compared to nonshock patients. Several novel approaches, including the use of L-NMNA and percutaneous ventricular-assist devices, are presently under investigation (61–63).

C. Late Clinical and Angiographic Outcomes

The initial clinical benefit of mechanical reperfusion is maintained at late follow-up (Fig. 4.5). Several studies have demonstrated a lower incidence of death and reinfarction in patients treated with primary PCI compared with thrombolytic therapy (43,44,64,65). Late angiographic outcomes are also significantly better with angioplasty. Of note, late infarct vessel reocclusion, which has an important impact on left ventricular remodeling, is significantly lower with angioplasty than thrombolysis (Fig. 4.6) (66–70). As discussed, the rates of restenosis and reocclusion have decreased with use of coronary stenting. Further improvements in late angiographic outcomes are anticipated with drug-eluting stent systems.

IV. LIMITATIONS OF PRIMARY PCI

A. The Importance of Microvascular Perfusion

Although primary PCI restores normal *epicardial* coronary artery flow in >90% of patients with acute myocardial infarction, a large number

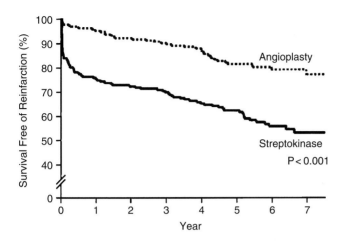

Figure 4.5 Kaplan-Meier curves for survival free of reinfarction in the angio-plasty and streptokinase groups during follow-up. The rate of survival free of reinfarction was higher in the group of 194 patients assigned to undergo angioplasty than in the group assigned to receive streptokinase. (From Ref. 65.)

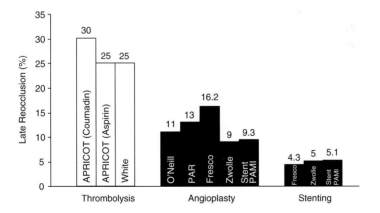

Figure 4.6 Late reocclusion of the infarct-related artery after thrombolytic therapy or primary angioplasty or stenting for acute myocardial infarction [APRICOT (66) = 3-month follow-up; White (68) = 1-year; PTCA & stent trials (9,29,30,32) = 6-month follow-up].

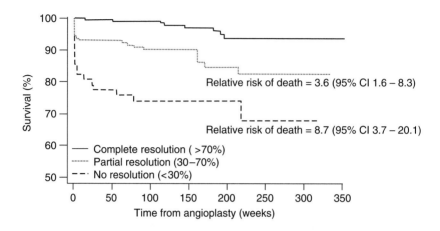

Figure 4.7 Relationship between extent of ST segment resolution and long-term outcome after primary angioplasty for acute myocardial infarction. (From Ref. 74.)

of these patients have suboptimal perfusion at a tissue level (71). Mechanisms contributing to poor *myocardial* perfusion are not well understood but are thought to include ischemia-induced microvascular damage, distal embolization, and reperfusion injury. Studies utilizing sensitive measures of myocardial perfusion, such as ST segment resolution, angiographic blush scores, contrast echocardiography and cardiac magnetic resonance imaging, have shown worse clinical outcomes in patients with poor tissue level flow (Fig. 4.7) (72–76). Accordingly, several pharmacological and mechanical approaches designed to enhance myocardial perfusion and improve myocardial salvage are under investigation.

Recent pharmacological therapies that have shown promise in clinical trials include adenosine, pexelizumab, and glucose-insulin-potassium (GIK). In the AMISTAD-2 trial, patients treated with high-dose adenosine had a smaller infarct size (11% vs. 26%; $p = 0.03$) (77). The COMMA trial evaluated the effect of pexelizumab, a novel C5 complement inhibitor, to reduce reperfusion injury (78). Although there was no difference in infarct size between study groups, there was a surprising mortality benefit in patients treated with pexelizumab bolus plus infusion. There has also been renewed interest in metabolic modulation using GIK since the results of the Zwolle trial were reported. Among patients without signs of heart failure (Killip I), there was a substantial reduction in mortality (1.2% vs. 4.2%; $p < 0.01$) (79). Further studies are being planned with both pexelizumab and GIK.

Mechanical approaches to improve myocardial perfusion include systemic hypothermia, hyperoxemic reperfusion, and devices to limit the effects of distal embolization (80,81). Experimental studies have demonstrated that mild hypothermia reduces metabolic demand in the risk region and limits infarct size. In the recently completed COOL-MI trial, hypothermia appeared to be beneficial in patients with anterior infarction if the heart was cooled adequately before reperfusion (82). Hyperoxemic reperfusion, utilizing intracoronary infusion of blood supersaturated with oxygen, also appears to be a promising adjunct therapy in myocardial infarction (AMI-HOT trial). Techniques to limit the effects of distal embolization include the use of thrombectomy devices and distal protection systems. Two studies have demonstrated that patients treated with adjunctive thrombectomy prior to stenting have a lower incidence of angiographic complications and improved ST segment resolution compared to patients treated without thrombectomy (83,84). Improved angiographic outcomes have also been reported with a filter-based distal protection system (85).

B. Improving the Availability of Mechanical Reperfusion

Although the use of mechanical reperfusion has increased over the last decade (Fig. 4.8), most patients with acute myocardial infarction are admitted to hospitals without facilities or trained personnel to perform primary PCI (86–88). Traditionally, fibrinolytic therapy has been the preferred first-line reperfusion strategy in these patients, although nearly 50% of patients are subsequently transferred to an invasive facility (87). Given the overwhelming advantages of mechanical reperfusion, particularly in high-risk patients, a number of strategies have evolved to optimize management of patients presenting to noninvasive centers. Of these new approaches, the patient transfer strategy has had the greatest impact on clinical practice patterns.

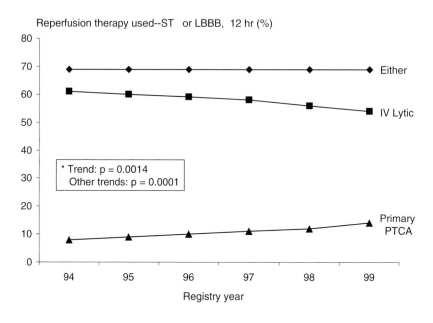

Figure 4.8 Temporal trends in the use of reperfusion therapy for patients with ST elevation myocardial infarction within 12 hours from symptom onset in the National Registry of Myocardial Infarction 1, 2 and 3 trials. (From Ref. 86.)

1. Patient Transfer for Primary PCI

Until recently, emergency transfer of patients with acute myocardial infarction was not recommended because of concern about the deleterious effect of delaying treatment on clinical outcomes and myocardial salvage. Six randomized trials have been conducted to determine the optimal reperfusion strategy in patients with acute myocardial infarction presenting to hospitals without invasive facilities (89–94). The largest of these were DANAMI-2 and PRAGUE-2 (93,94). Patients were treated either on-site with fibrinolysis (t-PA in DANAMI-2; streptokinase in PRAGUE-2) or transferred to an invasive center for emergency cardiac catheterization and coronary intervention when indicated. In both trials there was a dramatic reduction in the incidence of major adverse cardiac events at 30 days in the invasive groups (Fig. 4.9). It is important to note, however, that the door-to-treatment

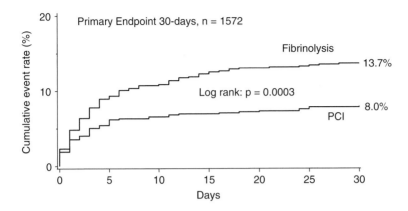

Figure 4.9   Incidence of the primary endpoint (death, myocardial infarction, and stroke) at 30 days in patients with STEMI treated on-site with fibrinolysis (t-PA) or transferred for cardiac catheterization and PCI. (From Ref. 93.)

time in both studies was <120 minutes despite the additional delay incurred during transportation (median time 115 minutes in DANAMI-2; 97 minutes in PRAGUE-2).

In a recent meta-analysis of the six randomized trials, patient transfer for primary PCI was associated with a 42% reduction in the composite endpoint (death/reinfarction/stroke), compared with a strategy of on-site thrombolysis (Fig. 4.10) (95). This was driven mainly by a reduction in the incidence of reinfarction (68% reduction) and stroke (56% reduction), but there was also a trend toward improved survival with PCI. Overall, these findings strongly support community wide adoption of a transfer strategy for mechanical reperfusion, as long as patient transfer can be accomplished within time intervals similar to those described in the randomized trials. The challenge now is to overcome logistical obstacles and replicate these impressive results in clinical practice.

2.   Primary PCI without Surgical Backup

An alternative approach is to perform primary PCI at centers without on-site cardiac surgery. Previous guidelines recommended that primary

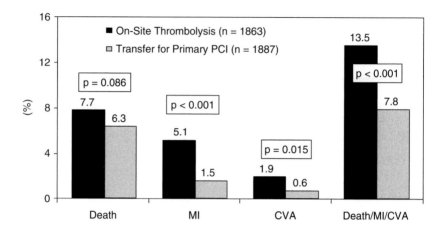

Figure 4.10 Meta-analysis of six randomized trials of transfer for primary angioplasty versus immediate thrombolysis for acute myocardial infarction. (From Ref. 95.)

angioplasty be performed only in centers with immediate surgical backup, in case the patient should require emergency bypass surgery because of unfavorable coronary anatomy or procedure-related complications. Coronary stents and glycoprotein IIb/IIIa inhibitors have dramatically improved the safety of primary PCI, so that emergency bypass surgery is now rarely needed. The Atlantic C-PORT trial, the only prospective study to evaluate the efficacy of mechanical reperfusion at hospitals without on-site surgery, randomized 451 patients to on-site PCI or thrombolysis (96). At 6 months the PCI group had a significantly lower incidence of the composite endpoint (death/myocardial infarction/stroke) than the t-PA group (12.4 vs. 19.9%; $p = 0.03$). Based on these findings, the ACC/AHA guidelines now acknowledge that primary PCI can be performed without on-site surgery, but the success of such a program is highly dependent on establishing rigorous standards and criteria to achieve these excellent outcomes (97,98).

3. Regionalization of Acute MI Care: The Heart Attack Center

In contradistinction to the community PCI approach, there has been growing interest in establishing regional centers of excellence to treat patients with acute myocardial infarction (99). Using this model, patients with suspected myocardial infarction would be transported to the nearest heart attack center, rather than the closest community hospital, in a system analogous to that used for trauma victims. Prehospital electrocardiographic diagnosis would facilitate initial patient triage and provide a mechanism for direct admission to the cardiac catheterization laboratory (100). Such a program, however, would require close cooperation between emergency medical services, community hospitals, and regional facilities to achieve these goals.

C. The Issue of Time to Reperfusion

In experimental studies, the relationship between the duration of coronary artery occlusion and extent of myocardial necrosis is unequivocal (101). Accordingly, the primary goal of reperfusion therapy is to restore blood flow in the infarct vessel as early as possible to salvage jeopardized myocardium and preserve ventricular function. Data from a number of randomized trials of thrombolytic therapy have confirmed this notion (102,103). In aggregate, these studies suggest that the mortality benefit of fibrinolytic therapy is strongly time dependent, with the greatest response observed in those patients presenting early after symptom onset.

In contrast, the relationship between time-to-treatment and clinical outcomes has been the subject of intense debate for patients undergoing mechanical reperfusion. This controversy has been fueled, in part, by the discordant results of clinical studies (104–110). Some reports have identified an association between time-to-reperfusion and survival, while others have found no clear relationship. Difficulty in interpretation of these observational data is further compounded by our inability to account for the dynamic nature of coronary occlusion in humans, failure to examine the importance of collateral circulation, differences in study design and analysis, and marked patient heterogeneity

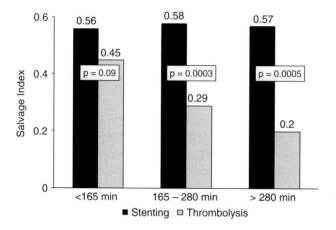

Figure 4.11 Myocardial salvage index according to tertiles of time-to-treatment interval. There was a time-dependent decrease of the salvage index in the thrombolysis group ($p = 0.03$) but not in the stenting group ($p = 0.59$) (From Ref. 111.)

depending on time to presentation. Notwithstanding these issues, the available data do suggest that efforts should be made to minimize the time-to-reperfusion during primary PCI, although the impact of treatment delay is less important than for patients treated with thrombolytic therapy. This effect may be explained, in part, by the observation that mechanical reperfusion, as opposed to fibrinolysis, results in significant myocardial salvage, independent of the time-to-treatment interval (Fig. 4.11) (111). Further, the impact of time-to-reperfusion during primary PCI appears to be closely related to the baseline risk profile (112,113). Notably, patients with cardiogenic shock or those stratified as "non-low risk" (using the TIMI criteria) do have a linear association between time-to-reperfusion and mortality and thus should be treated expeditiously (Figs. 4.12 and 4.13).

D. The Importance of Infarct Vessel Patency before PCI

Among patients undergoing primary PCI, spontaneous reperfusion (TIMI 3 flow) is observed in 10–20% of cases at initial angiography.

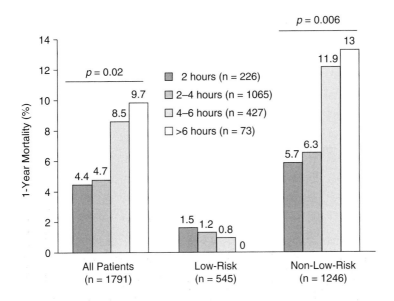

Figure 4.12 Relationship between symptom onset-to-balloon time and 1-year mortality according to the baseline risk profile (defined using the TIMI criteria). (From Ref. 112.)

These patients have a more favorable hospital course and long-term outcome than those presenting with an occluded infarct vessel (114,115). The importance of reperfusion before PCI has been high-lighted in two recent analyses from the PAMI group. Patients with normal epicardial flow at presentation were found to have better ventricular function, less heart failure, and lower early and late mortality. In fact, TIMI 3 grade flow before PCI was identified as an independent predictor of survival (odds ratio 2.1; $p = 0.04$), even when corrected for by postprocedural TIMI 3 flow (Fig. 4.14). Thus, early spontaneous reperfusion has an important salutary effect on clinical outcomes following primary PCI. These observations are consistent with pathophysiological mechanisms and suggest that early restoration of flow in the infarct vessel diminishes the extent of infarction. Moreover, an open artery also facilitates the interventional procedure, reducing catheterization-related complications and improving procedural success. These

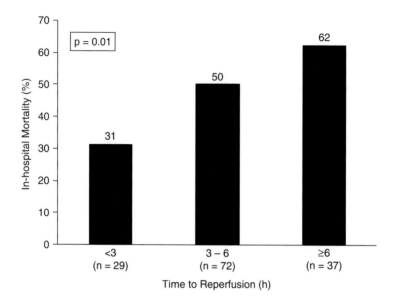

Figure 4.13 In-hospital mortality in patients with cardiogenic shock according to the time to reperfusion. Data are from the Moses Cone Hospital Registry. (From Ref. 113.)

observations have led to a rekindled interest in the potential synergy of a combined fibrinolytic and early invasive strategy. Whether this pharmacoinvasive reperfusion strategy will yield clinical benefit over primary PCI alone remains to be established in ongoing clinical trials (116).

V. CONCLUSION

Catheter-based reperfusion has emerged as the treatment of choice for patients with ST segment elevation myocardial infarction in centers with appropriate facilities and technical expertise. Contemporary data clearly demonstrate advantages of this strategy compared with thrombolytic therapy, particularly in patients at high risk. Although tremendous progress has been made in the last 10 years, many questions and

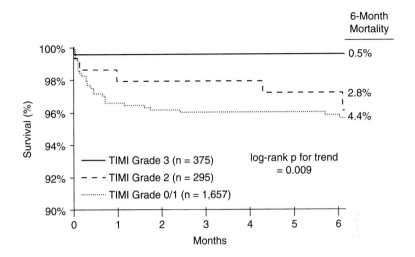

Figure 4.14 Cumulative survival (in-hospital plus late) after primary PTCA for acute myocardial infarction stratified by initial TIMI flow grade. Mortality is strongly correlated with TIMI flow before intervention. (From Ref. 115.)

challenges lie ahead. Notably, new therapeutic strategies are required to enhance myocardial perfusion following primary PCI. Most important, ongoing research will address methods to widen the availability of mechanical reperfusion in the community, particularly for high-risk patients admitted to hospitals without an interventional program.

REFERENCES

1. DeWood MA, Spores J, Notske R, et al. Prevalence of total coronary occlusion during the early hours of transmural myocardial infarction. N Engl J Med 1980; 303: 897–902.

2. Rentrop KP, Blanke H, Karsch KR. Acute myocardial infarction: intracoronary application of nitroglycerin and streptokinase: report of a prospective randomized trial. Clin Cardiol 1979; 2: 354–363.

3. Khaja F, Walton JA Jr, Brymer JF, et al. Intracoronary fibrinolytic therapy in acute myocardial infarction: report of a prospective randomized trial. N Engl J Med 1983; 308; 1305–1311.

4. Kennedy JW, Ritchie JL, Davis KB, et al. Western Washington randomized trial of intracoronary streptokinase in acute myocardial infarction. N Engl J Med 1983; 390: 1477–1482.

5. Rentrop KP, DeVivie ER, Karsch KR, et al. Acute coronary occlusion with impending infarction as an angiographic complication relieved by guide-wire recanalization. Clin Cardiol 1978; 1: 101–106.

6. Rentrop KP, Blanke H, Karsch KR, et al. Initial experience with transluminal recanalization of the recently occluded infarct-related coronary artery in acute myocardial infarction — comparison with conventionally treated patients. Clin Cardiol 1979; 2: 92–105.

7. Meyer J, Merx W, Schmitz H, et al. Percutaneous transluminal coronary angioplasty immediately after intracoronary streptolysis of transmural myocardial infarction. Circulation 1982; 66: 905–913.

8. Hartzler GO, Rutherford BD, McConahay DR, et al. Percutaneous transluminal coronary angioplasty with and without thrombolytic therapy for treatment of acute myocardial infarction. Am Heart J 1983; 106: 965–973.

9. O'Neill W, Timmis G, Bourdillon P, et al. A prospective randomized clinical trial of intracoronary streptokinase versus coronary angioplasty for acute myocardial infarction. N Engl J Med 1986; 314: 812–818.

10. Gruppo Italiano per lo Studio della Streptochinasi nell'Infarto Miocardico (GISSI). Effectiveness of intravenous thrombolytic treatment in acute myocardial infarction. Lancet 1986; 1: 397–402.

11. ISIS-2 Collaborative Group. Randomized trial of intravenous streptokinase, oral aspirin, both, or neither among 17,187 cases of suspected acute myocardial infarction. Lancet 1988; 2: 349–360.

12. Williams DO, Ruocco NA, Forman S, and the TIMI Investigators. Coronary angioplasty after recombinant tissue-type plasminogen activator in acute myocardial infarction: a report from the Thrombolysis in Myocardial Infarction (TIMI) trial. J Am Coll Cardiol 1987; 10: 45B–50B.

13. Topol EJ, Califf RM, George BS, et al. A randomized trial of immediate versus delayed elective angioplasty after intravenous tissue plasminogen activator in acute myocardial infarction. N Engl J Med 1987; 317: 581–588.

14. Simoons ML, Arnold AER, Betriu A, et al. Thrombolysis with t-PA in acute myocardial infarction: no beneficial effects of immediate PTCA. Lancet 1988; 1: 197–203.

15. The TIMI Research Group. Immediate vs. delayed catheterization and angioplasty following thrombolytic therapy for acute myocardial infarction: TIMI IIA results. JAMA 1988; 260: 2849–2858.

16. Holmes DR, Topol EJ. Reperfusion momentum: lessons learned from the randomized trials of immediate coronary angioplasty for myocardial infarction. J Am Coll Cardiol 1989; 14: 1572–1578.

17. The GUSTO Investigators. An international randomized trial comparing four thrombolytic strategies for acute myocardial infarction. N Engl J Med 1993; 329: 673–682.

18. Zijlstra F, de Boer MJ, Hoorntje JCA, et al. A comparison of immediate coronary angioplasty with intravenous streptokinase in acute myocardial infarction. N Engl J Med 1993; 328: 680–684.

19. Ribeiro EE, Silva LA, Carneiro R, et al. Randomized trial of direct coronary angioplasty versus intravenous streptokinase in acute myocardial infarction. J Am Coll Cardiol 1993; 22: 376–380.

20. Grinfeld L, Berrocal D, Belardi J, et al. Fibrinolytics vs. primary angioplasty in acute myocardial infarction (FAP): a randomized trial in a community hospital in Argentina. J Am Coll Cardiol 1996; 27 (suppl A): 222A.

21. Zijlstra F, Beukema WP, van't Hof AWJ, et al. Randomized comparison of primary coronary angioplasty with thrombolytic therapy in low risk patients with acute myocardial infarction. J Am Coll Cardiol 1997; 29: 908–912.

22. De Wood MA. Direct PTCA vs. intravenous t-PA in acute myocardial infarction: results from a prospective randomized trial. In: Proceedings from the Thrombolysis and Interventional Therapy in Acute Myocardial Infarction Symposium VI. Washington, DC: George Washington University Press, 1990: 28–29.

23. Grines CL, Browne KF, Marco J, et al. for the Primary Angioplasty in Myocardial Infarction Study Group. A comparison of immediate angioplasty with thrombolytic therapy for acute myocardial infarction. N Engl J Med 1993; 328: 673–679.

24. Gibbons RJ, Holmes DR, Reeder GS, et al. for the Mayo Coronary Care Unit and Catheterization Laboratory Groups. Immediate angioplasty compared with the administration of a thrombolytic agent followed by conservative treatment for myocardial infarction. N Engl J Med 1993; 328: 685–691.

25. Ribichini F, Steffenino G, Dellavalle A, et al. Comparison of thrombolytic therapy and primary coronary angioplasty with liberal stenting for inferior myocardial infarction with precordial ST-segment depression. Immediate and long-term results of a randomized study. J Am Coll Cardiol 1998; 32: 1687–1694.

26. Garcia E, Elizaga J, Perez-Castellano N, et al. Primary angioplasty versus systemic thrombolysis in anterior myocardial infarction. J Am Coll Cardiol 1999; 33: 605–611.

27. The Global Use of Stategies to Open Occluded Coronary Arteries in Acute Coronary Syndromes (GUSTO IIb) Angioplasty Substudy Investigators. A clinical trial comparing primary coronary angioplasty with tissue plasminogen activator for acute myocardial infarction. N Engl J Med 1997; 336: 1621–1628.

28. Rodriguez A, Bernardi V, Fernandez M, et al. on behalf of the GRAMI Investigators. In-hospital and late results of coronary stents versus conventional balloon angioplasty in acute myocardial infarction (GRAMI Trial). Am J Cardiol 1998; 81: 1286–1291.

29. Antoniucci D, Santoro GM, Bolognese L, et al. A clinical trial comparing primary stenting of the infarct-related artery with optimal primary angioplasty for acute myocardial infarction: results from the Florence Randomized Elective Stenting in Acute Coronary Occlusions (FRESCO) trial. J Am Coll Cardiol 1998; 31:1234–1239.

30. Suryapranata H, van't Hof AWJ, Hoorntje JC, et al. Randomized comparison of coronary stenting with balloon angioplasty in selected patients with acute myocardial infarction. Circulation 1998; 97: 2502–2505.

31. Saito S, Hosokawa G, Tanaka S, Nakamura S, for the PASTA Trial Investigators. Primary stent implantation is superior to balloon angioplasty in acute myocardial infarction: final results of the Primary Angioplasty versus Stent Implantation in Acute Myocardial Infarction (PASTA) trial. Cathet Cardiovasc Interven 1999; 48: 262–268.

32. Grines CL, Cox DA, Stone GW, et al. for the Stent Primary Angioplasty in Myocardial Infarction Study Group. Coronary angioplasty with or without stent implantation for acute myocardial infarction. N Engl J Med 1999; 341: 1949–1956.

33. Maillard L, Hamon M, Khalife K, et al. for the STENTIM-2 Investigators. A comparison of systematic stenting and conventional balloon angioplasty during primary percutaneous transluminal coronary angioplasty for acute myocardial infarction. J Am Coll Cardiol 2000; 35: 1729–1736.

34. Stone GW, Grines CL, Cox DA, et al. Comparison of angioplasty with stenting, with or without abciximab, in acute myocardial infarction. N Engl J Med 2002; 346: 957–966.

35. The EPIC Investigators. The use of a monoclonal antibody directed against the platelet glycoprotein IIb/IIIa receptor in high-risk coronary angioplasty. N Engl J Med 1994; 330: 956–961.

36. Lefkovits J, Ivanhoe RJ, Califf RM, et al. for the EPIC Investigators. Effects of platelet glycoprotein IIb/IIIa receptor blockade by a chimeric monoclonal antibody (abciximab) on acute and 6-month outcomes after percutaneous transluminal coronary angioplasty for acute myocardial infarction. Am J Cardiol 1996; 77: 1045–1051.

37. Brener SJ, Barr LA, Burchenal JEB, et al. on behalf of the ReoPro and Primary PTCA Organization and Randomized Trial (RAPPORT) Investigators. Randomized, placebo-controlled trial of platelet glycoprotein IIb/IIIa blockade with primary angioplasty for acute myocardial infarction. Circulation 1998; 98: 734–741.

38. Montalescot G, Barragan P, Wittenberg O, et al. for the ADMIRAL Investigators. Platelet glycoprotein IIb/IIIa inhibition with coronary stenting for acute myocardial infarction. N Engl J Med 2001; 344: 1895–1903.

39. Neumann FJ, Kastrati A, Schmitt C, et al. Effect of glycoprotein IIb/IIIa receptor blockade with abciximab on clinical and angiographic restenosis rate after the placement of coronary stents following acute myocardial infarction. J Am Coll Cardiol 2000; 35: 915–921.

40. Antoniucci D, Rodriguez A, Hempel A, et al. A randomized trial comparing primary infarct artery stenting with or without abciximab in acute myocardial infarction. J Am Coll Cardiol 2003; 42: 1879–1885.

41. Tcheng JE, Kandzari DE, Grines CL, et al. Benefits and risks of abciximab use in primary angioplasty for acute myocardial infarction. Circulation 2003; 108: 1316–1323.

42. Topol EJ, Neumann FJ, Montalescot G. A preferred reperfusion strategy for acute myocardial infarction. J Am Coll Cardiol 2003; 42: 1886–1888.

43. Keeley EC, Boura JA, Grines CL. Primary angioplasty versus intravenous thrombolytic therapy for acute myocardial infarction: a quantitative review of 23 randomised trials. Lancet 2003; 361: 13–20.

44. PCAT Collaborators. Primary coronary angioplasty compared with intravenous thrombolytic therapy for acute myocardial infarction: six-month follow up and analysis of individual patient data from randomized trials. Am Heart J 2003; 145: 47–57.

45. Cragg DR, Friedman HZ, Bonema JD, et al. Outcome of patients with acute myocardial infarction who are ineligible for thrombolytic therapy. Ann Intern Med 1991; 115: 173–177.

46. Zahn R, Schuster S, Schiele R, et al. Comparison of primary angioplasty with conservative therapy in patients with acute myocardial infarction and contraindications for thrombolytic therapy. Maximum Individual Therapy in Acute Myocardial Infarction (MITRA) Study Group. Cathet Cardiovasc Interv 1999; 46: 127–133.

47. Grzybowski M, Clements EA, Parsons L, et al. Mortality benefit of immediate revascularization of acute ST-segment elevation myocardial infarction in patients with contraindications to thrombolytic therapy. JAMA 2003; 290: 1891–1898.

48. Fibrinolytic Therapy Trialists (FTT) Collaborative Group. Indications for fibrinolytic therapy in suspected acute myocardial infarction: collaborative overview of early mortality and major morbidity results from all randomised trials of more than 1000 patients. Lancet 1994; 343: 311–322.

49. Lee KL, Woodlief LH, Topol EJ, et al. Predictors of 30-day mortality in the era of reperfusion for acute myocardial infarction. Results from an international trial of 41,021 patients. GUSTO-I Investigators. Circulation 1995; 91: 1659–1668.

50. Stone GW, Grines CL, Browne KF, et al. Predictors of in-hospital and 6-month outcome after acute myocardial infarction in the reperfusion era: The Primary Angioplasty in Myocardial Infarction (PAMI) trial. J Am Coll Cardiol 1995; 25: 370–377.

51. Holmes DR, White HD, Pieper KS, et al. Effect of age on outcome with primary angioplasty versus thrombolysis. J Am Coll Cardiol 1999; 33: 412–419.

52. DeGeare VS, Stone GW, Grines L, et al. Angiographic and clinical characteristics associated with increased in-hospital mortality in elderly patients with acute myocardial infarction undergoing percutaneous intervention: a pooled analysis of the primary angioplasty in myocardial infarction trials. Am J Cardiol 2000; 86: 30–34.

53. de Boer MJ, Ottervanger JP, van't Hof AW, et al. Reperfusion therapy in elderly patients with acute myocardial infarction: a randomized comparison of primary angioplasty and thrombolytic therapy. J Am Coll Cardiol 2002; 39: 1729–1732.

54. Peterson LR, Chandra NC, French WJ, et al. for the National Registry of Myocardial Infarction-2 Investigators. Reperfusion therapy in patients with acute myocardial infarction and prior coronary artery bypass graft surgery (National Registry of Myocardial Infarction-2). Am J Cardiol 1999; 84: 1287–1291.

55. Stone GW, Brodie BR, Griffin JJ, et al. for the Second Primary Angioplasty in Myocardial Infarction Trial (PAMI-2) Investigators. Clinical and angiographic outcomes in patients with previous coronary artery bypass graft surgery treated with primary balloon angioplasty for acute myocardial infarction. J Am Coll Cardiol 2000; 35: 605–611.

56. Labinaz M, Sketch MH, Ellis SG, et al. for the Global Utilization of Streptokinase and Tissue Plasminogen Activator for Occluded Coronary Arteries trial (GUSTO-I). Outcome of acute ST-segment elevation myocardial infarction in patients with prior coronary artery bypass surgery receiving thrombolytic therapy. Am Heart J 2001; 141: 469–477.

57. Suwaidi JA, Velianou JL, Berger PB, et al. Primary percutaneous coronary interventions in patients with acute myocardial infarction and prior coronary artery bypass grafting. Am Heart J 2001; 142: 452–459.

58. Nguyen TT, O'Neill WW, Grines CL, et al. One-year survival in patients with acute myocardial infarction and a saphenous vein graft culprit treated by primary angioplasty. Am J Cardiol 2003; 91: 1250–1254.

59. Prewitt RM, Gu S, Garber PJ, Ducas J. Marked systemic hypotension depresses coronary thrombolysis induced by intracoronary administration of recombinant tissue-type plasminogen activator. J Am Coll Cardiol 1992; 20: 1626–1633.

60. Hochman JS, Sleeper LA, Webb JG, et al. for the SHOCK Investigators. Early revascularization in acute myocardial infarction complicated by cardiogenic shock. N Engl J Med 1999; 341: 625–634.

61. Cotter G, Kaluski E, Blatt A, et al. L-NMMA (a nitric oxide synthase inhibitor) is effective in the treatment of cardiogenic shock. Circulation 2000; 101; 1358–1361.

62. Cotter G, Kaluski E, Milo O, et al. LINCS: L-NAME (a NO synthase inhibitor) in the treatment of refractory cardiogenic shock: a prospective randomized study. Eur Heart J 2003; 24: 1279–1281.

63. Thiele H, Lauer B, Hambrecht R, et al. Reversal of cardiogenic shock by percutaneous left atrial-to-femoral arterial bypass assistance. Circulation 2001; 104: 2917–2222.

64. Nunn CM, O'Neill WW, Rothbaum D, et al. for the Primary Angioplasty in Myocardial Infarction I study group. Long-term outcome after primary angioplasty: report from the Primary Angioplasty in Myocardial Infarction (PAMI-1) trial. J Am Coll Cardiol 1999; 33: 640–646.

65. Zijlstra F, Hoorntje JCA, de Boer MJ, et al. Long-term benefit of primary angioplasty as compared with thrombolytic therapy for acute myocardial infarction. N Engl J Med 1999; 341: 1413–1419.

66. Meijer A, Verheugt FWA, Werter CJPJ, et al. Aspirin versus coumadin in the prevention of reocclusion and recurrent ischemia after successful thrombolysis: a prospective placebo-controlled angiographic study. Results of the APRICOT study. Circulation 1993; 87: 1524–1530.

67. Veen G, de Boer MJ, Zijlstra F, Verheugt FWA. Improvement in three-month angiographic outcome suggested after primary angioplasty for acute myocardial infarction (Zwolle trial) compared with successful thrombolysis (APRICOT trial). Am J Cardiol 1999; 84: 763–767.

68. White HD, French JK, Hamer AW, et al. Frequent reocclusion of patent infarct-related arteries between four weeks and one year. Effects of antiplatelet therapy. J Am Coll Cardiol 1995; 25: 218–223.

69. Brodie BR, Stuckey TD, Kissling G, et al. Importance of infarct-related artery patency for recovery of left ventricular function and late survival after primary angioplasty for acute myocardial infarction. J Am Coll Cardiol 1996; 28: 319–325.

70. White HD, Cross DB, Elliot JM, Norris RM, Yee TW. Long-term prognostic importance of patency of the infarct-related coronary artery after thrombolytic therapy for acute myocardial infarction. Circulation 1994; 89: 61–67.

71. Ito H, Tomooka T, Sakai N, et al. Lack of myocardial perfusion immediately after successful thrombolysis. A predictor of poor recovery of left ventricular function in anterior myocardial infarction. Circulation 1992; 85: 1699–1705.

72. Gibson CM, Cannon CP, Murphy SA, et al. for the TIMI (Thrombolysis in Myocardial Infarction) study group. Relationship of TIMI myocardial perfusion grade to mortality after administration of thrombolytic drugs. Circulation 2000; 101: 125–130.

73. van't Hof AWJ, Liem A, Suryapranata H, et al., on behalf of the Zwolle Myocardial Infarction Study Group. Angiographic assessment of myocardial reperfusion in patients treated with primary angioplasty for acute myocardial infarction. Myocardial blush grade. Circulation 1998; 97: 2302–2306.

74. van't Hof AWJ, Liem A, de Boer MJ, Zijlstra F, for the Zwolle Myocardial Infarction Study Group. Clinical value of 12-lead electrocardiogram after successful reperfusion therapy for acute myocardial infarction. Lancet 1997; 350: 615–619.

75. Claeys MJ, Bosmans J, Veenstra L, et al. Determinants and prognostic implications of persistent ST-segment elevation after primary angioplasty for acute myocardial infarction. Importance of microvascular reperfusion injury on clinical outcome. Circulation 1999; 99: 1972–1977.

76. Wu KC, Zerhouni EA, Judd RM, et al. Prognostic significance of microvascular obstruction by magnetic resonance imaging in patients with acute myocardial infarction. Circulation 1998; 97: 765–772.

77. Ross A, on behalf of the AMISTAD-II Investigators. Acute Myocardial Infarction Study of Adenosine II. Presented at the Annual Scientific Session of the American College of Cardiology, Atlanta, GA, March 2002.

78. Granger CB, Maheffey KW, Weaver D, et al. Pexelizumab, an anti-C5 complement antibody, as adjunctive therapy to primary percutaneous coronary intervention in acute myocardial infarction. Circulation 2003; 108: 1184–1190.

79. van der Horst IC, Zijlstra F, van't Hof AWJ, et al. Glucose-insulin-potassium infusion in patients treated with primary angioplasty for acute myocardial infarction. J Am Coll Cardiol 2003; 42: 784–791.

80. Dixon SR, Whitbourn RJ, Dae MW, et al. Induction of mild systemic hypothermia with endovascular cooling during primary percutaneous coronary intervention for acute myocardial infarction. J Am Coll Cardiol 2002; 40: 1928–1934.

81. Dixon SR, Bartorelli AL, Marcovitz PA, et al. Initial experience with hyperoxemic reperfusion after primary angioplasty for acute myocardial infarction: results of a pilot study utilizing intracoronary aqueous oxygen therapy. J Am Coll Cardiol 2002; 39: 387–392.

82. O'Neill WW, on behalf of the COOL-MI Investigators. Cooling as an adjunct to primary PCI for acute myocardial infarction. Presented at Transcatheter Cardiovascular Therapeutics 2003, Washington, DC, September 2003.

83. Napodano M, Pasquetto G, Sacca S, et al. Intracoronary thrombectomy improves myocardial reperfusion in patients undergoing direct angioplasty for acute myocardial infarction. J Am Coll Cardiol 2003; 42: 1395–1402.

84. Lefevre T, Ludwig J, on behalf of the XAMINE ST Investigators. X-Sizer in AMI patients for Negligible Embolization and Optimal ST resolution. Presented at Transcatheter Cardiovascular Therapeutics 2003, Washington, DC, September 2003.

85. Limbruno U, Micheli A, de Carlo M, et al. Mechanical prevention of distal embolization during primary angioplasty. Safety, feasibility and impact on myocardial reperfusion. Circulation 2003; 108: 171–176.

86. Rogers WJ, Canto JG, Lambrew CT, et al. Temporal trends in the treatment of over 1.5 million patients with myocardial infarction in the US from 1990 through 1999. J Am Coll Cardiol 2000; 36: 2056–2063.

87. Rogers WJ, Canto JG, Barron HV, et al. for the investigators in the National Registry of Myocardial Infarction. Treatment and outcome of myocardial infarction in hospitals with and without invasive capability. J Am Coll Cardiol 2000; 35: 371–379.

88. Every NR, Parsons LS, Fihn SD, et al. for the MITI investigators. Long-term outcome in acute myocardial infarction patients admitted to hospitals with and without on-site cardiac catheterization facilities. Circulation 1997; 96: 1770–1775.

89. Vermeer F, Oude Ophuis AJM, vd Berg EJ, et al. Prospective randomised comparison between thrombolysis, rescue PTCA, and primary PTCA in patients with extensive myocardial infarction admitted to a hospital without PTCA facilities: a safety and feasibility study. Heart 1999; 82: 426–431.

90. Widimsky P, Groch L, Zelizko M, et al. on behalf of the PRAGUE Study Group Investigators. Multicentre randomized trial comparing transport to primary angioplasty vs. immediate thrombolysis vs. combined strategy for patients with acute myocardial infarction presenting to a community hospital without a catheterization laboratory. The PRAGUE Study. Eur Heart J 2000; 21: 823–831.

91. Grines CL, Westerhausen DR, Grines LL, et al. A randomized trial of transfer for primary angioplasty versus on-site thrombolysis in patients with high-risk myocardial infarction: the Air Primary Angioplasty in Myocardial Infarction Study. J Am Coll Cardiol 2002; 39: 1713–1719.

92. Bonnefoy E, Lapostolle F, Leizorovicz A, et al. Primary angioplasty versus prehospital fibrinolysis in acute myocardial infarction: a randomised study. Lancet 2002; 360: 825–829.

93. Andersen HR, Nielsen TT, Rasmussen K, et al. A comparison of coronary angioplasty with fibrinolytic therapy in acute myocardial infarction. N Engl J Med 2003; 349: 733–742.

94. Widimsky P, Budesinsky T, Vorac D, et al. Long distance transport for primary angioplasty vs. immediate thrombolysis in acute myocardial infarction. Final results of the randomized national multicentre trial — PRAGUE-2. Eur Heart J 2003; 94–104.

95. Dalby M, Bouzamondo A, Lechat P, Montalescot G. Transfer for primary angioplasty versus immediate thrombolysis in acute myocardial infarction. A meta-analysis. Circulation 2003; 108: 1809–1814.

96. Aversano T, Aversano LT, Passamani E, et al. Thrombolytic therapy vs. primary percutaneous coronary intervention for myocardial infarction in patients presenting to hospitals without on-site cardiac surgery. JAMA 2002; 287: 1943–1951.

97. Smith SC, Jr, Dove JT, Jacobs AK, et al. ACC/AHA guidelines for percutaneous coronary intervention: executive summary and recommendations: a report of the American College of Cardiology/American Heart Association Task Force on Practice Guidelines. J Am Coll Cardiol 2001; 37: 2215–2238.

98. Wharton TP, McNamara NS, Fedele FA, et al. Primary angioplasty for the treatment of acute myocardial infarction: experience at two community hospitals without cardiac surgery. J Am Coll Cardiol 1999; 33: 1257–1265.

99. Topol EJ, Kereiakes DJ. Regionalization of care for acute ischemic heart disease. Circulation 2003; 107: 1463–1466.

100. Canto JG, Rogers WJ, Bowlby LJ, et al. The prehospital electrocardiogram in acute myocardial infarction: is its full potential being realized? J Am Coll Cardiol 1997; 29: 498–505.

101. Reimer KA, Lowe JE, Rasmussen MM, Jennings RB. The wavefront phenomenon of ischemic cell death. I. Myocardial infarct size vs. duration of coronary occlusion in dogs. Circulation 1977; 56: 786–794.

102. Newby LK, Rutsch WR, Califf RM, et al. for the GUSTO-I Investigators. Time from symptom onset to treatment and outcomes after thrombolytic therapy. J Am Coll Cardiol 1996; 27: 1646–1655.

103. Goldberg RJ, Mooradd M, Gurwitz JH, et al. Impact of time to treatment with tissue plasminogen activator on morbidity and mortality following acute myocardial infarction (The Second National Registry of Myocardial Infarction). Am J Cardiol 1998; 82: 259–264.

104. Brodie BR, Stuckey TD, Wall TC, et al. Importance of time to reperfusion for 30-day and late survival and recovery of left ventricular function after primary angioplasty for acute myocardial infarction. J Am Coll Cardiol 1998; 32: 1312–1319.

105. Liem AL, van't Hof AWJ, Hoorntje JCA, et al. Influence of treatment delay on infarct size and clinical outcome in patients with acute myocardial infarction treated with primary angioplasty. J Am Coll Cardiol 1998; 32: 629–633.

106. Berger PB, Ellis SG, Holmes DR, et al. for the GUSTO-II Investigators. Relationship between delay in performing direct coronary angioplasty and early clinical outcome in patients with acute myocardial infarction. Results from the Global Use of Strategies to Open Occluded Arteries in Acute Coronary Syndromes (GUSTO-IIb) Trial. Circulation 1999; 100: 14–20.

107. Cannon CP, Gibson CM, Lambrew CT, et al. Relationship of symptom-onset-to-balloon time and door-to-balloon time with mortality in patients undergoing angioplasty for acute myocardial infarction. JAMA 2000; 283: 2941–2947.

108. Brodie BR, Stone GW, Morice MC, et al. Importance of time to reperfusion on outcomes with primary coronary angioplasty for acute myocardial infarction (results from the Stent Primary Angioplasty in Myocardial Infarction Trial). Am J Cardiol 2001; 88: 1085–1090.

109. Brodie BR, Stuckey TD, Hansen CJ, et al. Effect of treatment delay on outcomes in patients with acute myocardial infarction transferred from community hospitals for primary percutaneous coronary intervention. Am J Cardiol 2002; 89: 1243–1247.

110. Zijlstra F, Patel A, Jones M, et al. Clinical characteristics and outcome of patients with early (<2h), intermediate (2–4h) and late (>4h) presentation treated by primary coronary angioplasty or thrombolytic therapy for acute myocardial infarction. Eur Heart J 2002; 23: 550–557.

111. Schomig A, Ndrepepa G, Mehilli J, et al. Therapy-dependent influence of time-to-treatment interval on myocardial salvage in patients with acute myocardial infarction treated with coronary artery stenting or thrombolysis. Circulation 2003; 108: 1084–1088.

112. De Luca G, Suryapranata H, Zijlstra F, et al. Symptom-onset-to-balloon time and mortality in patients with acute myocardial infarction treated by primary angioplasty. J Am Coll Cardiol 2003; 42: 991–997.

113. Brodie BR, Stuckey TD, Muncy DB, et al. Importance of time-to-reperfusion in patients with acute myocardial infarction with and without cardiogenic shock treated with primary percutaneous coronary intervention. Am Heart J 2003; 145: 708–715.

114. Brodie BR, Stuckey TD, Hansen C, Muncy D. Benefit of coronary reperfusion before intervention on outcomes after primary angioplasty for acute myocardial infarction. Am J Cardiol 2000; 85: 13–18.

115. Stone GW, Cox D, Garcia E, et al. Normal flow (TIMI 3) before mechanical reperfusion therapy is an independent determinant of survival in acute myocardial infarction: analysis from the Primary Angioplasty in Myocardial Infarction trials. Circulation 2001; 104: 636–641.

116. Dauerman HL, Sobel BE. Synergistic treatment of ST segment elevation acute myocardial infarction with pharmacoinvasive recanalization. J Am Coll Cardiol 2003; 42:646–651.

II

The Evolution of Combination Therapy: Thrombolysis and PCI

5

Diminished Enthusiasm Reflecting Complications in Early Trials of Thrombolysis Followed by Coronary Intervention

**MATTHEW GUTIERREZ and
DAVID J. SCHNEIDER**

University of Vermont
Burlington, Vermont, U.S.A.

I. THE APPEAL OF COMBINING INVASIVE CORONARY INTERVENTION WITH THROMBOLYSIS

Results from the Thrombolysis in Myocardial Infarction (TIMI) I study confirmed that prompt myocardial reperfusion decreased mortality (1). Results of several large-scale trials before and after TIMI I were consistent in establishing that treatment with intravenously administered thrombolytic agents to recanalize infarct-related arteries decreased mortality in patients with ST elevation myocardial infarction (STEMI) (2,3). However, despite the obvious benefits of thrombolysis, 30-day mortality in the GISSI-2 and ISIS-3 trials was as high as 8–10% (4,5). Because early restoration of myocardial blood flow was shown to preserve left ventricular function and reduce mortality, subsequent trials were designed to identify treatment regimens designed to induce more rapid and persistent recanalization.

The GUSTO trial demonstrated that treatment of patients within 6 hours after onset of symptoms with the combination of a clot-selective thrombolytic agent [recombinant tissue type plasminogen activator (t-PA)] plus conjunctive treatment with aspirin and intravenous unfractionated heparin resulted in 30-day mortality of 6.3% (6). An angiographic substudy demonstrated that patency of the infarct-related artery was not the sole determinant of outcome. Restoration of normal coronary flow after thrombolysis was found to be critical in lowering mortality (7). Thus, angiographic analysis demonstrated that both induction of culprit artery patency and the extent of restoration of flow were determinants of outcome.

The importance of restoration of flow was demonstrated further in a pooled analysis involving more than 5000 patients (8). A 30-day mortality of approximately 9% was seen with the absence of restoration of flow (TIMI 0 flow) or with residual, marked limitation of flow (TIMI 1 flow), whereas mortality was 3–4% in patients with fully restored apparently normal flow (TIMI 3 flow). Lenderink and colleagues found that mortality in patients who had induction of vessel patency but reduced blood flow (TIMI 2 flow) was similar to that in patients with TIMI 0 or 1 flow and lower than that in patients with TIMI 3 flow (8). Thus, angiographic results demonstrated that optimal outcome can be achieved only when flow is reestablished promptly and fully in the infarct artery.

II. LIMITATIONS OF THROMBOLYSIS ALONE

When treatment is initiated with intravenous rt-PA within 6 hours after onset of symptoms, patency of the infarct artery is evident in 70–90% of patients (7,9). Considered from the opposite perspective, intravenous administration of a clot-selective thrombolytic agent does not induce patency in the infarct-related artery in at least 10–20% of patients. This may reflect the severity of the underlying occlusion, the nature of the vulnerable plaque, the age of the thrombus, and other factors. Approximately 40% of patients do not exhibit normal (TIMI 3) flow in the region of supply of the infarct artery 90 minutes after thrombolysis (7,8). These observations support the concept that a combination of percutaneous coronary intervention plus coronary thrombolysis may be optimal for restoring and maintaining flow in the infarct-related artery.

Two observations that led many early investigators to combine pharmacological reperfusion with PCI were the recurrence of symptoms of ischemia and reocclusion of the infarct-related artery after initially successful thrombolysis. In one report, 65% of patients with a subtotal occlusion and 48% who had exhibited manifestations of reperfusion had recurrent ischemic events (10). Those with recurrent ischemia had higher in-hospital mortality (11). Accordingly, investigators postulated that the combination of subsequent PCI with pharmacological reperfusion might achieve early restoration of flow combined with more effective and more persistent normalization of flow as well as a decreased incidence of reocclusion and reinfarction.

III. EARLY EXPERIENCE WITH COMBINED THROMBOLYSIS AND OBLIGATORY, SUBSEQUENT CORONARY INTERVENTION

Three influential studies explore thrombolysis followed by obligatory coronary intervention compared with thrombolysis alone. These results diminished enthusiasm for a combined approach. A primary objective of one component of the TIMI II trial (TIMI IIa) was to determine whether early invasive management after acute STEMI would improve outcome (12). Patients eligible for enrollment in TIMI II were those with symptoms of less than 4 hours in duration and electrocardiographic manifestations of acute STEMI. All patients were treated with intravenous recombinant t-PA. In addition to t-PA, patients were treated with contemporary conjunctive and adjunctive therapy that included aspirin, unfractionated heparin, and intravenous lidocaine for a minimum of 24 hours. Within 1 hour after onset of infusion of t-PA, patients were given a bolus of 5000 units of unfractionated heparin in addition to a continuous infusion of 1000 units per dose to induce a 1.5- to 2-fold increase in the activated partial thromboplastin time (aPPT) compared with control. The rate of administration of the heparin infusion was decreased before left heart catheterization was performed, and heparin was continued at full dosage for a total of 5 days after the procedure.

In the TIMI IIa trials, patients were randomized to immediate cardiac catheterization and coronary intervention or to cardiac catheterization and intervention performed within 18–48 hours (12). The primary endpoint was the predischarge left ventricular ejection fraction. A similar ejection fraction was seen in those randomized to delayed catheterization (49%) and to immediate catheterization and PIC (50.3%). However, the incidence of bleeding and the requirement for urgent coronary bypass surgery were greater in those randomized to early coronary intervention. Mortality and the incidence of reinfarction were similar in those treated with either the early invasive or the more conservative strategy. Accordingly, no relatively greater clinical benefit was seen with immediate compared with delayed PCI. However, immediate PCI was associated with a greater risk of bleeding and a greater need for emergency coronary bypass surgery. Similar results were obtained in the contemporaneous European Cooperative trial (13). The concordance of results in these two influential trials led to virtual abandonment of enthusiasm for a combined approach.

However, the potential value of the combination of pharmacological thrombolysis plus PCI was revisited in the SWIFT (Should We Intervene Following Thrombolysis) trial (14). In the SWIFT trial patients were treated with anistreplase. The primary endpoint was death or reinfarction after 12 months (14). This multicenter, randomized trial involved 800 patients with acute STEMI from the United Kingdom and Ireland. Conjunctive therapy included 1000 units per hour of unfractionated heparin (started 4–6 hours after thrombolysis) and warfarin (initiated at the discretion of each physician). Adjunctive treatment was the timolol (unless contraindicated). Of the 397 patients treated with early intervention, 169 patients underwent PTCA and 59 had surgery. After 12 months, the incidences of death and reinfarction were similar in each group. In addition, the incidence of angina and the left ventricular ejection fraction were similar in those treated with coronary intervention or undergoing then conventional care.

The European Cooperative Study had already randomized 367 patients with acute STEMI (13). t-PA had been administered to eligible patients within 5 hours after onset of symptoms. Conjunctive therapy had included aspirin (250 mg) and unfractionated heparin (5000 units bolus plus 1000 units per hour infusion). Treatment with warfarin was allowed at the discretion of the treating physician. In those randomized to subsequent early intervention, angiography had been performed as promptly as possible (within 165 minutes), and PCI had been performed when anatomy was appropriate.

The trial was terminated prematurely by the data and safety monitoring committee. The enzymatic estimates of the infarct size and left ventricular function were similar in those treated with early intervention compared with conservative therapy. However, a trend toward increased mortality was apparent in the intervention group. Analysis of coronary patency and residual stenosis at the time of discharge showed no difference in the incidence of patency. However, less residual stenosis was seen in the intervention group. The incidences of bleeding and blood transfusion were higher (41% and 10%) in the invasive strategy group.

Thus, overall in the three trials that assessed the potential benefit of a strategy in which thrombolysis was combined with PCI in the treatment of acute STEMI, no evidence of clinical benefit attributable to prompt PCI following thrombolysis was apparent. By contrast, complications occurred at an increased frequency. None of the trials had been powered to assess an impact on mortality. However, the lack of improvement in left ventricular ejection fraction, enzymatic estimate of infarct size, or the incidence of reinfarction was deemed to be discouraging. Moreover, the lack of apparent benefit was associated with an increased risk of bleeding.

IV. MECHANISMS POTENTIALLY RESPONSIBLE FOR THE LACK OF BENEFIT SEEN IN EARLY TRIALS COMBINING PCI WITH PHARMACOLOGICAL THROMBOLYSIS

At first glance, the lack of benefit associated with the combination of mechanical reperfusion with initial thrombolysis calls into question the potential benefit of a pharmacoinvasive approach. Nevertheless, improved outcomes had been seen consistently in those patients who exhibited full restoration of myocardial blood flow (7,8). Because myocyte necrosis begins within minutes after coronary occlusion, any increased delay entailed in implementation of a combined approach may have contributed to the lack of improvement in left ventricular function when PCI was combined with administration of thrombolytic agents. However, some benefit has been associated with restoration of myocardial blood flow even when it is induced more than 4 hours after the onset of symptoms. Thus, delays in the restoration of flow are not likely to have been the sole determinant of a lack of benefit (2–6). In addition, PCI offered promise of diminishing the risk of reocclusion. Accordingly, the combination of initial thrombolysis and subsequent PCI was thought by many to remain attractive. The high incidence of complications encountered in the early studies of a combined approach has been obviated by technological and pharmacologic advances. Thus, they do not militate against pharmacoinvasive therapy today.

Milavetz and colleagues found that reperfusion was a critical determinant of benefit during the first 2 hours after onset of symptoms and that the restoration of normal blood flow remained a key determinant even when symptoms had begun more than 2 hours earlier (15). Unfortunately, most patients with an acute STEMI will seek medical attention only after more than 2 hours after onset of symptoms. Accordingly, the lack of clinical benefit associated with a combined approach used in the early trials is likely to have been a function of then contemporary limitations of pharmacological therapy, limitations of coronary intervention, and "cultural" and "system" limitations precluding prompt initiation of treatment.

No marked incremental improvement in the overall success of thrombolysis alone has been identified after that seen with the initial GUSTO study. The GUSTO study demonstrated conclusively that a clot-sensitive thrombolytic agent (t-PA) plus immediate implementation of conjunctive antithrombotic therapy with unfractionated heparin and aspirin was associated with a remarkably low 30-day mortality. Newer agents such as tenectoplase (TNK) are easy to administer because of their longer elimination half-life. However, clinical trials with such agents have not demonstrated a reduced 30-day incidence of death (16,17). Despite the development of novel antiplatelet and anti-coagulant agents, their combination with clot-selective thrombolytic agents has not reduced 30-day mortality (18,19). This may reflect, in part, the insensitivity of mortality as an endpoint in studies comparing diverse, novel, thrombolytic regimens and agents. Regardless, the excellent results obtained in TIMI IIa, the European Cooperative trial, and SWIFT have been difficult to surpass.

In contrast to pharmacological reperfusion, advances in the success and safety of PCI have occurred during the period following TIMI IIa, the European Cooperative Study, and SWIFT. The availability of intracoronary stents has improved substantially restoration of blood flow with PIC (20,21). The Controlled Abciximab and Device Investigation to Lower Late Angioplasty Complications (CADILLAC) investigators found that the incidence of the primary endpoint of a 6-month incidence of death, reinfarction, disabling stroke, and ischemia-driven revascularization of the target vessel was reduced from 20 to 11.5% when PCI was performed with stents rather than balloon angioplasty. Thus, one mechanism that may have contributed to the lack of efficacy of a combined approach in the earlier trials was the then obligatory use of balloon angioplasty without the availability of intracoronary stents, bailout catheters, and other recently developed devices.

The development of novel and powerful antiplatelet agents has improved outcomes after PCI. In the CADILLAC trial, the use of a glycoprotein IIb-IIIa inhibitor improved outcome in those treated with either balloon angioplasty or an intracoronary stent (21). Similarly, treatment with clopidogrel, a thienopyridine, decreases the incidence of adverse events after PCI (22,23). Neither thienopyridines nor glycoprotein IIb-IIIa antagonists were available at the time the early trials designed to test the potential clinical efficacy of a combined approach were performed.

In addition to a lack of clinical benefit, a greater incidence of bleeding complications was seen in early trials of pharmacoinvasive treatment. Both technological advances and improvement in pharmacological therapy have been shown to reduce the incidence of complications attributable to bleeding after PCI. Technological advances now permit performance of PCI with smaller-diameter catheters that are likely to decrease the subsequent risk of bleeding. Results in the EPILOG study demonstrated that the dosage of heparin is a critical determinant of the incidence of bleeding (24). Thus, heparin was likely to have contributed to the high incidence of bleeding complications in the early trials designed to evaluate a combined approach in treatment of STEMI.

V. SUMMARY AND CONCLUSIONS

Pharmacoinvasive treatment of STEMI is predicated on the observation that both the time or onset of reperfusion and the extent of restoration of flow in the infarct-related artery and consequent myocardial perfusion are determinants of outcome. Results from early trials such as TIMI IIa, the European Cooperative Study, and SWIFT failed to support the value of a combined approach as judged from endpoints such as recurrent myocardial infarction or improved left ventricular ejection fraction. In addition, an increase in the incidence of bleeding complications was seen. The lack of benefit is likely to have been related to the lack of availability of intracoronary stents and limitations in then contemporaneous pharmacological therapy including the lack of availability of powerful antiplatelet agents such as glycoprotein IIb-IIIa inhibitors and thienopyridines. The high incidence of bleeding is likely to have been related to the larger-diameter catheters and the high dosages of heparin that were employed. As discussed in subsequent chapters, the picture is very different today.

REFERENCES

1. Dalen JE, Gore JM, Braunwald E, Borer J, Goldberg RJ, Passamani ER, Forman S, Knatterud G. Six- and twelve-month follow-up of the phase I Thrombolysis in Myocardial Infarction (TIMI) trial. Am J Cardiol 1988;62:179–185.

2. GISSI Investigators. Effectiveness of intravenous thrombolytic treatment in acute myocardial infarction. Group Italiano per lo Studio della Streptochinasi nell'Infarto Miocardico (GISSI). Lancet 1986;1:397– 402.

3. ISIS-2 Investigators. Randomised trial of intravenous streptokinase, oral aspirin, both, or neither among 17,187 cases of suspected acute

myocardial infarction: ISIS-2. ISIS-2 (Second International Study of Infarct Survival) Collaborative Group. Lancet 1988;2:349–360.

4. GISSI-2 Investigators. GISSI-2: a factorial randomized trial of alteplase versus streptokinase and heparin versus no heparin among 12,490 patients with acute myocardial infarction. Gruppo Italiano per lo Studio della Sopravvivenza nell'Infarto Miocardico. Lancet 1990; 336:65–71.

5. ISIS-3 Investigators. ISIS-3: a randomized comparison of streptokinase vs. tissue plasminogen activator vs. anistreplase and of aspirin plus heparin vs. aspirin alone among 41,299 cases of suspected acute myocardial infarction. ISIS-3 (Third International Study of Infarct Survival) Collaborative Group. Lancet 1992;339:753–770.

6. The GUSTO Investigators. An international randomized trial comparing four thrombolytic strategies for acute myocardial infarction. N Eng J Med 1993;329:673–682.

7. The GUSTO Angiographic Investigators. The effects of tissue plasminogen activator, streptokinase, or both on coronary-artery patency, ventricular function, and survival after acute myocardial infarction. N Engl J Med 1993; 329:1615–1622.

8. Lenderink T, Simoons ML, Van Es GA, Van de Werf F, Verstraete M, Arnold AE. Benefit of thrombolytic therapy is sustained throughout five years and is related to TIMI perfusion grade 3 but not grade 2 flow at discharge. The European Cooperative Study Group. Circulation 1995;92:1110–1116.

9. Neuhaus KL, Feuerer W, Jeep-Tebbe S, Niederer W, Vogt A, Tebbe U. Improved thrombolysis with a modified dose regimen of recombinant tissue-type plasminogen activator. J Am Coll Cardiol 1989;14:1566–1569.

10. Schaer DH, Leiboff RH, Katz RJ, Wasserman AG, Bren GB, Varghese PJ, Ross AM. Recurrent early ischemic events after thrombolysis for acute myocardial infarction. Am J Cardiol 1987;59:788–792.

11. Stone GW, Grines CL, Browne KF, Marco J, Rothbaum D, O'Keefe J, Hartzler GO, Overlie P, Donohue B, Chelliah N, Timmis GC, Ronald Vlietsra R, Puchrowicz-Ochocki R, O'Neill WW, Marco J. Implications of recurrent ischemia after reperfusion therapy in acute myocardial

infarction: a comparison of thrombolytic therapy and primary angioplasty. J Am Coll Cardiol 1995;26:66–72.

12. The TIMI Research Group. Immediate versus delayed catheterization
and angioplasty following thrombolytic therapy for acute myocardial
infarction. JAMA 1988;260:2849–2858.

13. de Bono DP. The European Cooperative Study Group trial of intravenous recombinant tissue-type plasminogen activator (rt-PA) and conservative therapy versus rt-PA and immediate coronary angioplasty. J
Am Coll Cardiol 1988;12:20A–23A.

14. The SWIFT Investigators. SWIFT trial of delayed elective intervention
v conservative treatment after thrombolysis with anistreplase in acute
myocardial infarction. SWIFT (Should We Intervene Following
Thrombolysis?) Trial Study Group. BMJ 1991;302:555–560.

15. Milavetz JJ, Giebel DW, Christian TF, Schwartz RS, Holmes DR Jr,
Gibbons RJ. Time to therapy and salvage in myocardial infarction. J
Am Coll Cardiol 1998;31:1246–1251.

16. GUSTO III Investigators. A comparison of reteplase with alteplase for
acute myocardial infarction. N Engl J Med 1997;337:1118–1123.

17. ASSENT II Investigators. Single-bolus tenecteplase compared with
front-loaded alteplase in acute myocardial infarction: the ASSENT-2
double-blind randomized trial. Assessment of the Safety and Efficacy
of a New Thrombolytic Investigators. Lancet 1999;354:716–722.

18. Topol EJ, GUSTO V Investigators. Reperfusion therapy for acute myocardial infarction with fibrinolytic therapy or combination reduced
fibrinolytic therapy and platelet glycoprotein IIb/IIIa inhibition: the
GUSTO V randomized trial. Lancet 2001;357:1905–1914.

19. Assessment of the Safety and Efficacy of a New Thrombolytic Regimen
(ASSENT)-3 Investigators. Efficacy and safety of tenecteplase in combination with enoxaparin, abciximab, or unfractionated heparin: the
ASSENT-3 randomised trial in acute myocardial infarction. Lancet
2001;358:605–613.

20. Suryapranata H, van't Hof AW, Hoorntje JC, de Boer MJ, Zijlstra F.
Randomized comparison of coronary stenting with balloon angioplasty
in selected patients with acute myocardial infarction. Circulation 1998;
97:2502–2505.

21. Stone GW, Grines CL, Cox DA, Garcia E, Tcheng JE, Griffin JJ, Guagliumi G, Stuckey T, Turco M, Carroll JD, Rutherford BD, Lansky AJ, Controlled Abciximab and Device Investigation to Lower Late Angioplasty Complications (CADILLAC) Investigators. Comparison of angioplasty with stenting, with or without abciximab, in acute myocardial infarction. N Engl J Med 2002;346:957–966.

22. Mehta SR, Yusuf S, Peters RJ, Bertrand ME, Lewis BS, Natarajan MK, Malmberg K, Rupprecht H, Zhao F, Chrolavicius S, Copland I, Fox KA, Clopidogrel in Unstable Angina to Prevent Recurrent Events Trial (CURE) Investigators. Effects of pretreatment with clopidogrel and aspirin followed by long-term therapy in patients undergoing percutaneous coronary intervention: the PCI-CURE study. Lancet 2001;358: 527–533.

23. Steinhubl SR, Berger PB, Mann JT III, Fry ET, DeLago A, Wilmer C, Topol EJ, CREDO Investigators. Clopidogrel for the reduction of events during observation. Early and sustained dual oral antiplatelet therapy following percutaneous coronary intervention: a randomized controlled trial. JAMA 2002;288:2411–2420.

24. The EPILOG Investigators. Platelet glycoprotein IIb/IIIa receptor blockade and low-dose heparin during percutaneous coronary revascularization. N Engl J Med 1997;336:1689–1696.

6

The Rebirth of Interest in Pharmacoinvasive Therapy in the Stent Era

JACQUELINE SAW

Vancouver General Hospital
University of British Columbia
Vancouver, British Columbia, Canada

DAVID J. MOLITERNO

University of Kentucky
Lexington, Kentucky, U.S.A.

I. INTRODUCTION

Acute myocardial infarction (MI) occurs in approximately 540,000 patients yearly in the United States, of whom approximately one third ultimately die (1). The critical component to ensure preservation of myocardial function involves prompt restoration of coronary arterial flow at both the epicardial and microvascular levels. Reperfusion strategies have evolved utilizing potent antiplatelet, anticoagulation, and thrombolytic therapies, or mechanical approaches including percutaneous coronary intervention (PCI), intra-aortic balloon pump support, and emergent coronary artery bypass surgery. The combination of an antiplatelet and thrombolytic strategy together with mechanical revascularization for acute ST elevation myocardial infarction (STEMI) has recently gained widespread interest. This combined approach to STEMI is especially attractive given the availability of more potent and specific pharmaceuticals and technologically advanced interventional devices. In this chapter we will discuss how pharmacoinvasive reperfusion for STEMI has gained momentum in our current era of percutaneous coronary interventions.

II. THROMBOLYSIS

Rupture of a vulnerable atherosclerotic plaque is the most common trigger of thrombus formation in the coronary vasculature that results in an acute MI. The primary composition of thrombus consists of cross-linked fibrin with entrapped cellular elements. The body's intrinsic fibrinolytic system utilizes plasmin, a nonspecific protease, to digest the meshwork of fibrin clot into fibrinogen degradation productions. In order to be active, plasmin needs to undergo a single peptide bond cleavage from plasminogen. Furthermore, once formed, plasmin catalyzes additional plasminogen conversion into plasmin. Currently available thrombolytic agents are serine protease plasminogen activators that directly or indirectly convert plasminogen to plasmin. These thrombolytic agents differ in fibrin selectivity and half-life duration.

Since the introduction of thrombolytic agents for acute MI treatment in 1958, more than 200,000 patients have been studied in randomized controlled trials. The conglomerate data indicate a significant reduction of mortality with these agents that is inversely proportional and strongly dependent on the time to treatment (2) (Fig. 6.1). Indeed, 50% mortality reduction was achieved when thrombolytic therapy was administered within the first hour of pain onset (the golden hour), as shown in the MITI (Myocardial Infarction and Triage) (3), EMIP (European Myocardial Infarction Project) (4), GISSI-1 (Gruppo Italiano per lo Studio della Streptochinasi nell'Infarto Miocardico) (5), and ISIS-2 (Second International Study of Infarct Survival) (6) trials (Fig. 6.2). This mortality benefit declines to about 25% when thrombolytics were given up to 12 hours after pain onset (7–10), but no benefit beyond 12 hours of pain onset was demonstrated (9,10) (Figs. 6.1 and 6.2). It is estimated that 10 additional lives could be saved per 1000 patients for every hour that treatment was initiated earlier (11).

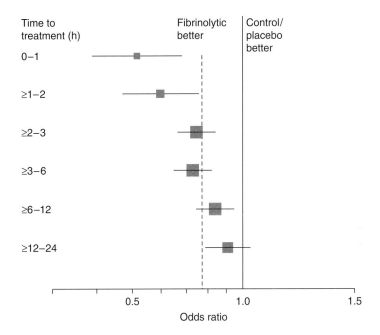

Figure 6.1 Effect of thrombolytic therapy on 35-day mortality according to time treatment delay. (From Ref. 2.)

Nevertheless, despite prompt thrombolytic therapy, only 50–60% of STEMI patients achieve complete restoration of epicardial coronary flow [Thrombolysis in Myocardial Infarction (TIMI) grade 3] at 90 minutes (12,13). Achievement of this TIMI 3 flow milestone is pivotal in improving long-term survival. For example, an angiographic substudy of GUSTO-1 (Global Utilization of Streptokinase and Tissue Plasminogen Activator for Occluded Coronary Arteries Trial) showed that TIMI 3 flow with thrombolytic therapy reduced 30-day mortality (hazard ratio 0.57) compared to TIMI grade 0–2 flows, with persistence of benefit to 2 years (hazard ratio 0.39) (Fig. 6.3) (14). Furthermore, restoration of TIMI myocardial perfusion (TMP), TMP 3, occurs in only a quarter of STEMI patients who receive thrombolysis (15). Similar to epicardial flow, better myocardial perfusion is associated with improved survival (Fig. 6.4) (15). The achievement of both TIMI 3 flow

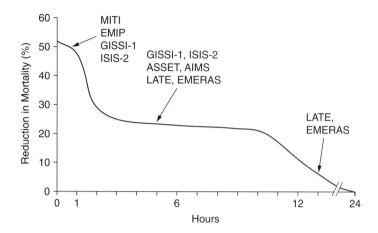

Figure 6.2 Percent mortality reduction as a function of the elapsed time between symptom onset and initiation of thrombolytic therapy. (From Ref. 35.)

and TMP 3 grade is associated with the lowest 30-day mortality (0.7%), compared with 10.9% for TIMI 0–1 and TMP 0–1 grades ($p < 0.001$) (15) (Fig. 6.5). Unfortunately, this ideal combination of epicardial and myocardial perfusion was attained in only ~18% of patients receiving thrombolysis (15). Moreover, there is a risk of reocclusion following thrombolytic therapy, necessitating conjunctive therapies with anti-platelet and antithrombin agents, all of which increase the risk of intracerebral hemorrhage.

III. PRIMARY PERCUTANEOUS CORONARY INTERVENTION

The limitations of thrombolytic therapy for STEMI led to the increasing dominance of the mechanical revascularization strategy, primary PCI. To date, more than 20 randomized trials involving more than 8000 patients have compared primary PCI with thrombolysis. A meta-analysis of these trials convincingly showed that primary angioplasty reduced short-term death (7% vs. 9%; $p = 0.0002$), nonfatal reinfarction (3% vs. 7%; $p = 0.0004$), and stroke (1% vs. 2%; $p = 0.0004$) (16).

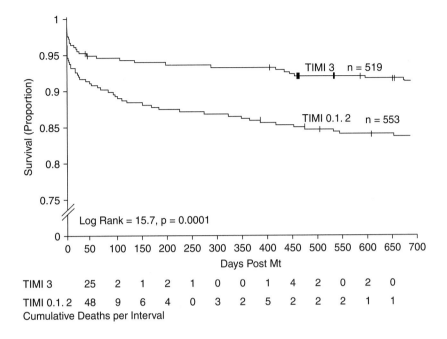

Figure 6.3 Achievement of TIMI 3 flow with thrombolytic therapy is associated with lower mortality at 30 days, with persistent benefit to 2 years, compared with lower-grade TIMI flows (0–2). (From Ref. 14.)

More than 90% of patients achieve TIMI 3 flow with primary PCI (17,18); however, normal myocardial perfusion was attained in only ~30% of patients despite TIMI 3 flow (19). Similar to thrombolytic therapy, the presence of normal epicardial and myocardial perfusion was associated with the best clinical outcomes. Among patients for whom TIMI 3 flow was restored, 1-year survival was 6.8% in the presence of normal myocardial blush, 13.2% with reduced myocardial blush, and 18.3% with absent myocardial blush ($p = 0.0004$) (Fig. 6.6) (19). Therefore, adjunctive aggressive pharmacotherapy (antiplatelet, antithrombotic, and fibrinolytic therapies) that could improve myocardial perfusion, further supplementing mechanical revascularization, will provide additive benefit to patients with STEMI. Furthermore, there is often a time delay from the door to balloon, which, compounded

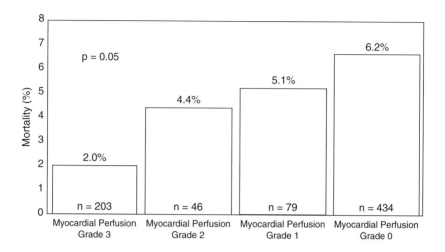

Figure 6.4 Relationship between myocardial perfusion grade and 30-day mortality. (From Ref. 15.)

with the lack of universal catheterization laboratories makes the strategy of pharmacoinvasive reperfusion (20) very attractive. The potential advantages of this combined approach include a reduction of the time delay inherent with purely mechanical approaches to reperfusion as well as improving myocardial perfusion. This strategy may particularly benefit centers where an invasive laboratory is not available and transfer to a tertiary center is required.

IV. PHARMACOINVASIVE THERAPY FOR STEMI

Early studies combining balloon angioplasty and antecedent thrombolytic therapy showed no clinical benefit and demonstrated higher mortality, reinfarction and bleeding events (21–23). (These trials are discussed in detail in Chapter 5.) Since the 1980s, the advances of percutaneous devices (especially coronary stents), potent antiplatelet agents [thienopyridines and glycoprotein (GP) IIb/IIIa inhibitors], and fibrin-specific bolus-injection thrombolytic agents may render these early studies no longer relevant. Several recent randomized trials have

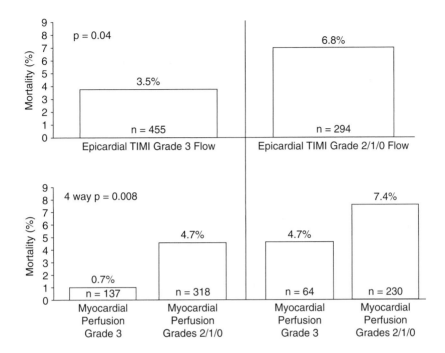

Figure 6.5   Relationship of epicardial TIMI flow and myocardial perfusion grade to 30-day mortality with thrombolytic therapy. (From Ref. 15.)

demonstrated the benefit of GP IIb/IIIa blockade and coronary stents in the setting of STEMI (24–27). The rebirth of interest in the combined approach can be traced to three contemporary pharmacoinvasive studies: PACT (Plasminogen-activator Angioplasty Compatibility Trial) (28), SPEED (Strategies for Patency Enhancement in the Emergency Department) (29), and TIMI 10B–14 (30).

PACT was a multicenter, randomized, double-blind, placebo-controlled study which enrolled 606 STEMI patients to rt-PA (IV 50 mg bolus over 3 min) or placebo (28). Patients then underwent immediate angiography (median time 98 min following hospital arrival) to determine patency of the infarct artery. Patients who had TIMI 0–2 flow underwent "rescue" (patients who received rt-PA) or primary (patients who received placebo) angioplasty, whereas those who had TIMI 3 flow

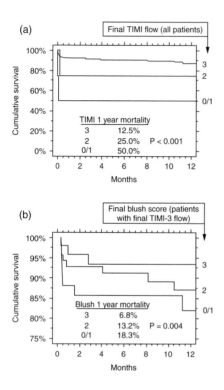

Figure 6.6 Cumulative survival (a) after primary angioplasty according to TIMI flow (b), and according to myocardial perfusion in the presence of TIMI 3 flow. (From Ref. 19.)

were given a second dose of the assigned study drug (angioplasty usually deferred). All patients received IV heparin (5000 u bolus, 1000 u/h infusion) for at least 48 hours; abciximab was administered to 5% of patients. Coronary stenting was used in 26% of patients who required PCI. TIMI 3 flow was present on initial angiography in 33% of patients who received rt-PA versus 15% of placebo patients ($p < 0.001$). Rescue angioplasty and primary angioplasty restored TIMI 3 flow in 77% and 79% of patients, respectively. Those who had TIMI 3 flow on arrival to the catheterization laboratory had better convalescent ejection fraction (62.4%) compared with later mechanical restoration (ejection fraction

57.9%) ($p = 0.004$). Furthermore, there was no difference in adverse events between rt-PA and placebo groups, irrespective of angioplasty procedures. Therefore, the PACT study showed that half-dose thrombolytic therapy followed by rescue angioplasty (if TIMI 3 flow was not initially achieved) is a feasible and safe strategy.

SPEED was a randomized trial comparing abciximab with or without varying doses of reteplase in STEMI patients presenting within 6 hours of chest pain onset (29). In the first dose-ranging phase of the trial, 304 patients were randomized to receive abciximab (0.25 mg/kd bolus, 0.125 µg/kg/min infusion for 12 h) with reteplase (5 U, 7.5 U, 10 U, 5 + 2.5 U, or 5 + 5 U boluses), or no reteplase. In the second dose-confirmation phase, 223 patients were randomized to full-dose reteplase (10 + 10 U) or abciximab with reduced-dose reteplase (5 + 5 U). All patients received aspirin and IV heparin (70 U/kg for those receiving full-dose reteplase, 40 U/kg for reduced-dose reteplase). The primary endpoint evaluated the incidence of TIMI 3 flow at 60–90 minutes in both phases. Coronary angiography was performed without delay after reperfusion therapy began, and PCI was performed at the interventionalist's discretion. There were 323 patients (61%) who underwent early PCI; this group was compared to 162 patients who did not undergo PCI. The clinical success rate (30-day freedom from death, reinfarction, or urgent revascularization for severe ischemia) was 85.4% for patients who underwent facilitated PCI and 70.4% for those who did not ($p < 0.001$) (Fig. 6.7). Patients who underwent early PCI had a lower rate of reinfarction, urgent revascularization, and transfusions (Fig. 6.8). Before PCI, only 66.3% of patients had TIMI 2–3 flow, but following early PCI this proportion increased to 97.6% ($p < 0.001$). Patients receiving combination therapy of abciximab and reduced-dose reteplase had the highest rate of TIMI 3 flow (47%) at 60 minutes, compared with those receiving abciximab alone (24.3%) or reteplase alone (39.3%) ($p = 0.05$ across the three groups). Post-PCI TIMI 3 flow was not different among the three groups ($p = 0.23$). There was also a trend toward improved 30-day clinical outcomes of death, MI, and urgent revascularization in the combination arm (5.9%), compared with abciximab alone (8.1%) or reteplase alone (7.1%). Therefore, this study showed that the combination strategy of abciximab with reduced-dose reteplase improved TIMI 3 flow in the infarct artery at 60–90 minutes

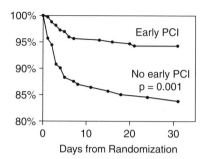

Figure 6.7 Freedom from the composite of death, reinfarction, or urgent revascularization at 30 days for patients who underwent early PCI (top line) or not (bottom line) in the SPEED trial. (From Ref. 29.)

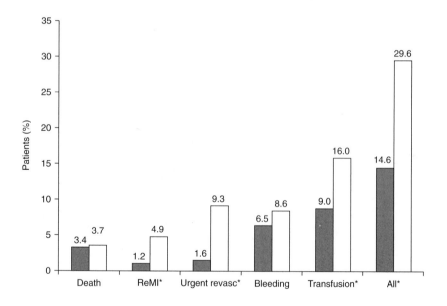

Figure 6.8 Major adverse events and bleeding complications in ST elevation MI patients undergoing early PCI ($n = 323$, black bars) compared with those who did not undergo early PCI ($n = 162$, white bars) in the SPEED trial. * Denotes $p < 0.05$. (From Ref. 29.)

after initiation of reperfusion therapy. Furthermore, early PCI was shown to be safe and effective compared with those who did not undergo PCI, irrespective of thrombolytic combination with GP IIb/IIIa blockade.

The results from SPEED are dramatically different from the earlier balloon angioplasty trials (21–23). These studies are performed about a decade apart, and there have been significant technological advances for both interventional techniques and pharmaceutical agents. Together with increased operator experience, the routine use of coronary stents, improved guide catheters, and coronary wires and balloons has led to improvements in technical and clinical success with PCI. The use of smaller-diameter catheters allows smaller sheath sizes that also help to reduce bleeding complications. The use of coronary stents decreases not only restenosis but also subacute thrombosis and reinfarction. In the setting of acute STEMI, the CADILLAC (Controlled Abciximab and Device Investigation to Lower Late Angioplasty Complications) trial clearly showed that coronary stenting reduced the 6-month primary endpoint of death, MI, revascularization, or disabling stroke compared with angioplasty alone (11.5% vs. 20.0%; $p < 0.001$) (26). In this regard, coronary stents were used in approximately 80% of patients undergoing early PCI in SPEED.

Greater comprehension of antithrombotic agents in the past decade has also led to utilization of lower-dose heparin as well as point-of-care monitoring devices, further decreasing bleeding rates. Furthermore, the introduction of GP IIb/IIIa inhibitors was a major development for PCI, especially for high-risk patients with acute coronary syndromes. Specifically, abciximab has been shown to be beneficial in several randomized primary PCI trials. In a pooled analysis of five published primary PCI trials, abciximab reduced 30-day death, MI, or target vessel revascularization compared with placebo (4.8% vs. 8.8%) (24–27,31,32) and also reduced death and MI at 6 months (31). The specific thrombolytic agent used in SPEED, reteplase, may also have contributed to the improved outcomes. Reteplase is given as a bolus injection without weight adjustment, thus simplifying and enabling earlier administration. Reteplase has also been shown to achieve greater TIMI 3 flow at 90 minutes compared with a front-loaded regimen of alteplase (59.9% vs. 45.2%; $p = 0.01$) (33), although the 30-day mortality rate was not different between these two regimens in the GUSTO-III trial (7.5% reteplase, 7.2% alteplase; $p = 0.54$) (34).

In a combined analysis of the TIMI 10B and TIMI 14 trials, Schweiger et al. reported similar beneficial outcomes with early PCI following acute STEMI (30). The TIMI 10B study randomized 841 STEMI patients to single bolus tenecteplase (30, 40, or 50 mg over 5–10 s) or standard front-loaded alteplase (accelerated over 90 min), whereas the TIMI 14 study randomized 834 STEMI patients to either standard alteplase or one of three experimental strategies (abciximab alone, abciximab with reduced-dose alteplase, or abciximab with reduced-dose streptokinase). All patients underwent angiography 90 minutes after initiation of reperfusion therapy. Treatment with PCI was left to the discretion of the operators. Rescue PCI was defined as performance of PCI 90–150 minutes after initiation of reperfusion for patients with TIMI 0–1 flow; adjunctive PCI was defined as performance of PCI after 90–150 minutes for TIMI 2–3 flow; and delayed PCI was defined as PCI >150 minutes after the start of pharmacological treatment. Overall, 56% of patients in TIMI 10B and 67% in TIMI 14 underwent PCI during hospitalization. Among patients with TIMI 0–1 flow at 90 minutes, those treated with rescue PCI had a lower mortality (6% vs. 17%; $p = 0.01$) and lower rate of death or recurrent MI (8% vs. 19%; $p = 0.01$) at 30 days compared with those who did not undergo PCI. In a multivariate logistic regression analysis, patients with TIMI 3 flow at 90 minutes were less likely to experience death or MI at 30 days if they underwent adjunctive or delayed PCI compared to those who did not undergo PCI (odds ratio 0.46; $p = 0.02$) (Fig. 6.9). Therefore, data from these studies are congruent with SPEED, reiterating that early PCI following thrombolytic or combined thrombolytic with GP IIb/IIIa blockade is safe and effective for patients with acute STEMI.

V. UPCOMING PHARMACOINVASIVE STUDIES

With the promising data from the aforementioned studies, several ongoing phase III studies are now evaluating the utility of facilitated PCI (combined GP IIb/IIIa blockade with reduced-dose thrombolytic therapy) for acute STEMI. These include FINESSE (Facilitated INtervention with

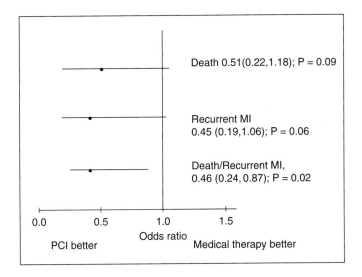

Figure 6.9   Odds ratio plot with 95% confidence intervals comparing 30-day outcomes in acute ST elevation MI patients with TIMI 3 flow at 90 minutes who underwent PCI (adjunctive or delayed) versus those who did not undergo PCI (medical therapy) in the TIMI 10B and 14 trials. (From Ref. 30.)

Enhanced reperfusion Speed to Stop Events) and ASSENT-4 (Fourth Assessment of the Safety and Efficacy of a New Thrombolytic). (The design of these studies will be reviewed in detail in Chapter 8.) The rebirth of interest in the pharmacoinvasive reperfusion strategy has already led to randomized trials testing this concept. SIAM-3 (Southwest German Interventional Study in Acute Myocardial Infarction-3) was a multicenter, randomized trial comparing early PCI after thrombolytic therapy to a strategy of thrombolysis with subsequent outpatient PCI at 2 weeks after lytics. This 162-patient trial demonstrated a significant benefit for the pharmacoinvasive reperfusion strategy as opposed to the more conservative thrombolytic arm. The nearly 50% reduction in the 6-month combined endpoint (ischemic events, death, reinfarction, target lesion revascularization 25.6% vs. 50.6%; $p = 0.001$) did not come at a cost of significantly increased bleeding with PCI performed on average 3.5 hours after initiation of thrombolytic therapy

(36). Other small to moderate-sized European study results have also been reported in a preliminary fashion and again echo the safety and possible increased efficacy of pharmacoinvasive reperfusion as compared to stand-alone thrombolysis or primary PCI. Ultimately, the results of large randomized trials such as FINESSE and ASSENT-4 will determine whether or not pharmacoinvasive reperfusion can indeed overcome the limitations inherent in the separated treatment options of thrombolysis and primary PCI.

VI. CONCLUSIONS

The practice of thrombolytic therapy and PCI in exclusion of each other for patients with acute STEMI has limitations, which thus prompted initial trials of a combination strategy. Unfortunately, early trials in the 1980s demonstrated harm and lack of clinical efficacy with this combined approach, which understandably propagated concerns such that the American College of Cardiology published guidelines labeling this approach as Class IIb in the management of acute STEMI patients. However, despite this recommendation, routine PCI for patent vessels following thrombolytic therapy is commonly performed in the United States. This approach is now partially condoned with the promising data from the SPEED, TIMI 10B, and TIMI 14 trials. Data from these studies reassured to clinicians that combining pharmacotherapy (with aggressive antiplatelet and reduced-dose thrombolytics) with an early invasive PCI approach is safe and probably efficacious with modern techniques, equipment, and pharmaceuticals (37). In a related issue, should all patients who received thrombolytic therapy undergo routine angiography after perceived clinical reperfusion? While this remains a contentious topic, at least proponents of an early invasive strategy now have more contemporary trials, albeit nonrandomized, to corroborate their decisions.

However, these trials are still limited by their methodology and designs. This includes the lack of randomization of early PCI versus no PCI in the trials investigating varying doses of thrombolytic and GP IIb/IIIa blockade.To remove selection bias and prove the increased efficacy of the pharmacoinvasive approach, only ongoing pharmocoinvasive trials can fully address the effectiveness of this combined strategy.

REFERENCES

1. American Heart Association. Heart Disease and Stroke Statistics — 2003 Update. Dallas, TX: American Heart Association; 2002.

2. Boersma E, Maas AC, Deckers JW, Simoons ML. Early thrombolytic treatment in acute myocardial infarction: reappraisal of the golden hour. Lancet 1996;348:771–775.

3. Weaver WD, Cerqueira M, Hallstrom AP, et al. Prehospital-initiated vs. hospital-initiated thrombolytic therapy. The Myocardial Infarction Triage and Intervention Trial. JAMA 1993;270:1211–1216.

4. The EMIP Group. Pre-hospital thrombolytic therapy in patients with suspected acute myocardial infarction. N Engl J Med 1993;329: 383–389.

5. Gruppo Italiano per lo Studio della Streptochinasi nell'Infarto Miocardico (GISSI). Effectiveness of intravenous thrombolytic treatment in acute myocardial infarction. Lancet 1986;1:397–402.

6. Second International Study of Infarct Survival Collaborative Group. Randomized trial of intravenous streptokinase, oral aspirin, both, or neither among 17,187 cases of suspected acute myocardial infarction: ISIS-2. Lancet 1988;2:349–360.

7. AIMS Trial Study Group. Effect of intravenous APSAC on mortality after acute myocardial infarction: preliminary report of a placebo-controlled clinical trial. Lancet 1988;1:545–549.

8. Wilcox RG, von der Lippe G, Olsson CG, Jensen G, Skene AM, Hampton JR. Trial of tissue plasminogen activator for mortality reduction in acute myocardial infarction. Anglo-Scandinavian Study of Early Thrombolysis (ASSET). Lancet 1988;2:525–530.

9. Wilcox R, for the LATE Steering Committee. Late assessment of thrombolytic efficacy with alteplase 6–24 hours after onset of acute myocardial infarction. Lancet 1993;342:759–766.

10. Estudio Multicentrico Estreptoquinasa Republicas de America del Sur (EMERAS) Collaborative Group. Randomized trial of late thrombolysis in patients with suspected acute myocardial infarction. Lancet 1993;342: 767–772.

11. Cannon CP, Antman EM, Walls R, Braunwald E. Time as an adjunctive agent to thrombolytic therapy. J Thromb Thrombolysis 1994;1:27–34.

12. GUSTO Angiographic Investigators. The effects of tissue plasminogen activator, streptokinase, or both on coronary artery patency, ventricular function, and survival after acute myocardial infarction. N Engl J Med 1993;329:1615–1622.

13. Smalling RW, Bode C, Kalbfleisch J, et al. More rapid, complete, and stable coronary thrombolysis with bolus administration of reteplase compared with alteplase infusion in acute myocardial infarction. RAPID Investigators. Circulation 1995;91:2725–2732.

14. Ross AM, Coyne KS, Moreyra E, et al. Extended mortality benefit of early postinfarction reperfusion. GUSTO-I Angiographic Investigators. Global Utilization of Streptokinase and Tissue Plasminogen Activator for Occluded Coronary Arteries Trial. Circulation 1998;97:1549–1556.

15. Gibson CM, Cannon CP, Murphy SA, et al. Relationship of TIMI myocardial perfusion grade to mortality after administration of thrombolytic drugs. Circulation 2000;101:125–130.

16. Keeley EC, Boura JA, Grines CL. Primary angioplasty versus intravenous thrombolytic therapy for acute myocardial infarction: a quantitative review of 23 randomised trials. Lancet 2003;361:13–20.

17. Zijlstra F, de Boer MJ, Hoorntje JC, Reiffers S, Reiber JH, Suryapranata H. A comparison of immediate coronary angioplasty with intravenous streptokinase in acute myocardial infarction. N Engl J Med 1993;328:680–684.

18. Nunn CM, O'Neill WW, Rothbaum D, et al. Long-term outcome after primary angioplasty: report from the primary angioplasty in myocardial infarction (PAMI-I) trial. J Am Coll Cardiol 1999;33:640–646.

19. Stone GW, Peterson MA, Lansky AJ, Dangas G, Mehran R, Leon MB. Impact of normalized myocardial perfusion after successful angioplasty in acute myocardial infarction. J Am Coll Cardiol 2002;39:591–597.

20. Dauerman HL, Sobel BE. Synergistic treatment of ST segment elevation myocardial infarction with pharmacoinvasive recanalization. J Am Coll Cardiol 2003; 46: 646–651.

21. Topol EJ, Califf RM, George BS, et al. A randomized trial of immediate versus delayed elective angioplasty after intravenous tissue plasminogen activator in acute myocardial infarction. N Engl J Med 1987;317:581–588.

22. Simoons ML, Arnold AE, Betriu A, et al. Thrombolysis with tissue plasminogen activator in acute myocardial infarction: no additional benefit from immediate percutaneous coronary angioplasty. Lancet 1988;1:197–203.

23. SWIFT trial of delayed elective intervention v conservative treatment after thrombolysis with anistreplase in acute myocardial infarction. SWIFT (Should We Intervene Following Thrombolysis?) Trial Study Group. BMJ 1991;302:555–560.

24. Brener S, Barr L, Burchenal J, et al. Randomized, placebo-controlled trial of platelet glycoprotein IIb/IIIa blockade with primary angioplasty for acute myocardial infarction. Circulation 1998;98:734–741.

25. Montalescot G, Barragan P, Wittenberg O, et al. Platelet glycoprotein IIb/IIIa inhibition with coronary stenting for acute myocardial infarction. N Engl J Med 2001;344:1895–1903.

26. Stone G, Grines C, Cox D, et al. Comparison of angioplasty with stenting, with or without abciximab, in acute myocardial infarction. N Engl J Med 2002;346:958–966.

27. Antoniucci D, Rodriguez A, Hempel A, et al. A randomized trial comparing primary infarct artery stenting with or without abciximab in acute myocardial infarction. J Am Coll Cardiol 2003;42:1879–1885.

28. Ross AM, Coyne KS, Reiner JS, et al. A randomized trial comparing primary angioplasty with a strategy of short-acting thrombolysis and immediate planned rescue angioplasty in acute myocardial infarction: the PACT trial. PACT investigators. Plasminogen-Activator Angioplasty Compatibility Trial. J Am Coll Cardiol 1999;34:1954–1962.

29. Herrmann HC, Moliterno DJ, Ohman EM, et al. Facilitation of early percutaneous coronary intervention after reteplase with or without abciximab in acute myocardial infarction: results from the SPEED (GUSTO-4 Pilot) Trial. J Am Coll Cardiol 2000;36:1489–1496.

30. Schweiger MJ, Cannon CP, Murphy SA, et al. Early coronary intervention following pharmacological therapy for acute myocardial infarction (the combined TIMI 10B-TIMI 14 experience). Am J Cardiol 2001;88:831–836.

31. Topol EJ, Neumann FJ, Montalescot G. A preferred reperfusion strategy for acute myocardial infarction. J Am Coll Cardiol 2003;42:1886–1889.

32. Neumann FJ, Kastrati A, Schmitt C, et al. Effect of glycoprotein IIb/IIIa receptor blockade with abciximab on clinical and angiographic restenosis rate after the placement of coronary stents following acute myocardial infarction. J Am Coll Cardiol 2000;35:915–921.

33. Bode C, Smalling RW, Berg G, et al. Randomized comparison of coronary thrombolysis achieved with double-bolus reteplase (recombinant plasminogen activator) and front-loaded, accelerated alteplase (recombinant tissue plasminogen activator) in patients with acute myocardial infarction. The RAPID II Investigators. Circulation 1996;94: 891–898.

34. A comparison of reteplase with alteplase for acute myocardial infarction. The Global Use of Strategies to Open Occluded Coronary Arteries (GUSTO III) Investigators. N Engl J Med 1997;337:1118–1123.

35. Lincoff AM, Topol EJ. Illusion of reperfusion. Does anyone achieve optimal reperfusion during acute myocardial infarction? Circulation 1993;88:1361–1374.

36. Scheller B, Hennen B, Hammer B, Walle J, Hofer C, Hilpert V, Winter H, Nickenig G, Bohm M. Beneficial effects of immediate stenting after thrombolysis in acute myocardial infarction. J Am Coll Cardiol 2003;46:634–641.

37. Dauerman HL. The early days after ST elevation acute myocardial infarction: reconsidering the delayed invasive approach. J Am Coll Cardiol 2003;42:420–423.

7

Pharmacological Developments Likely to Enhance the Benefits of Pharmacoinvasive Therapy

**ELLIOTT M. ANTMAN and
EUGENE BRAUNWALD**

Brigham and Women's Hospital
Boston, Massachusetts, U.S.A.

Timely reperfusion of jeopardized myocardium is the most effective means of restoring the balance between myocardial oxygen supply and demand in patients with ST elevation myocardial infarction (STEMI) (1,2). Two distinct approaches to reperfusion, pharmacologic and catheter-based, have been intensively studied and are widely utilized worldwide. However, such a dichotomous approach has a number of deficiencies (3). In addition to oversimplifying a complex science, it fails to emphasize adequately the role of ancillary treatments critical to the success or failure of a reperfusion strategy and limits the development of creative approaches that combine the two reperfusion strategies.

Contemporary concepts of ideal reperfusion reach beyond restoration of full antegrade flow (TIMI grade 3 flow) in the epicardial infarct artery. The goal of reperfusion in STEMI is to improve perfusion in

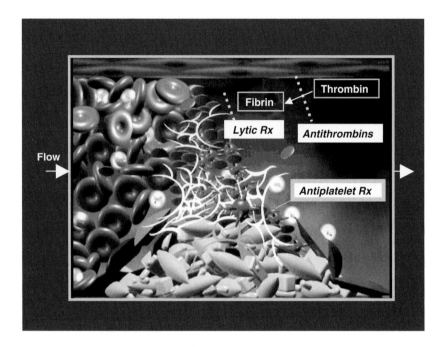

Figure 7.1 Schematic diagram of longitudinal view of infarct artery with superimposed major components of pharmacological reperfusion regimen. The high-risk or vulnerable plaque is shown at the bottom with disrupted cap. The contents of the plaque are exposed to the bloodstream with resultant activation of platelets (conversion of flat elements to spiked elements) and initiation of the coagulation cascade. Fibrin strands (white curvilinear arcs) are formed. Pharmacological reperfusion regimens consist of a fibrinolytic (plasminogen activator), an antithrombin, and an antiplatelet agent.

the zone of infarcting myocardium (4). Of note, the process of reperfusion, although beneficial in terms of myocardial salvage, may also come at a cost in the form of reperfusion injury.

Many of the pharmacological developments that are designed to enhance reperfusion have overlapping goals. Notable advances include improvements in each of the three major components of a pharmacological reperfusion regimen: fibrinolytics, antithrombins, and antiplatelets (Fig. 7.1). The antithrombin and antiplatelet advances have also improved catheter-based reperfusion approaches. Less dramatic in terms of success has been the development of agents to minimize reperfusion injury. As suggested by the term pharmacoinvasive therapy, introduced by Dauerman and Sobel, it is now appropriate to consider a more global strategy of reperfusion for STEMI that provides an effective and safe means of initiating timely pharmacological reperfusion to be buttressed subsequently by percutaneous coronary intervention (PCI) for optimal early and long-term outcomes (5).

I. FIBRINOLYTICS

The fibrinolytic agents currently available and under investigation are enzymatic plasminogen activators, which directly or indirectly expose the active catalytic center of plasmin. The efficacy of various fibrinolytic agents has generated considerable controversy. It is now established that the relatively fibrin-specific agent alteplase t-PA is associated with a mortality advantage over streptokinase because a higher proportion of patients achieve early (90-min) TIMI grade 3 flow in the infarct artery (6–8). Variants of t-PA have been constructed with the intention of developing an improved fibrinolytic in terms of efficacy and safety (Fig. 7.2). These variants have altered pharmacokinetic or functional properties that yield several desirable features: prolonged clearance from the circulation (permitting administration as a single or double bolus), enhanced fibrin specificity, and increased resistance to plasminogen activator inhibitor (PAI-1) (9).

Bolus fibrinolytics offer the distinct advantages of ease of administration and a reduced potential for dosing errors. Clinical trials indicate, however, that they are not superior to t-PA with respect to impact on mortality (10–13). Several important lessons were learned during the development of bolus fibrinolytics. As with the original development of t-PA, the dose of the fibrinolytics is fundamental to identification of a safe regimen. Thus, an unacceptably high rate of intracranial hemorrhage (ICH) of 1.89% occurred with 150 mg of t-PA, whereas it was reduced to 0.54% with a dose of 100 mg (6). Phase 2 experience with tenecteplase tissue-plasminogen activator (TNK) suggested that weight adjustment was important to reduce bleeding risk (11,14–16).

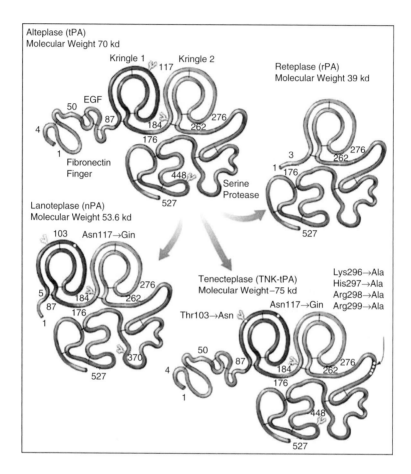

Figure 7.2 Molecular structure of alteplase (t-PA), lanoteplase (n-PA), reteplase (r-PA), and tenecteplase (TNK). Streptokinase is the least fibrin-specific thrombolytic agent in clinical use; the progressive increase in relative fibrin specificity for the various thrombolytics is shown at the bottom.

Adequately sized phase 2 trials are essential to proper dose selection for phase 3 trials and then establishing the appropriate clinical dose.

For both conventional and bolus fibrinolytic agents, it is now clear that conjunctive antithrombin and antiplatelet agents play a pivotal role not only in determining efficacy but also in the risk of bleeding. Despite the well-intentioned goal of increasing fibrinolytic efficacy, excessive dosing with an antithrombin is associated with an increased risk of bleeding, especially ICH (17).

For elderly patients, the decision to administer a fibrinolytic and selection of the dose and conjunctive agents are particular problems. Younger patients (<55 years) achieve a greater relative risk reduction (26%) in mortality with fibrinolysis compared to placebo than do elderly patients (4% relative risk reduction in patients >75 years) (18). However, the higher absolute mortality in the elderly results in a similar absolute risk difference compared with the young, translating into about 10 lives saved per 1000 patients treated with fibrinolysis regardless of age. Against this mortality advantage of fibrinolysis, one must weigh the increased risk of ICH in the elderly (19,20). The concept of a dose reduction of the fibrinolytic for the elderly is an appealing one. The modest impact of weight adjustment may be helpful in thin elderly patients but is probably not sufficient to compensate for the reduced clearance of fibrinolytics and conjunctive agents in elderly patients of all body weights. We propose a "75% rule" in which patients over the age of 75 receive 75% of the dose of a fibrinolytic agent; this awaits prospective testing.

Traditionally, fibrinolytics have been assessed by their ability to improve flow in the infarct artery according to the TIMI grading system (21). Only in studies in which a pretreatment coronary arteriogram documented occlusion of the culprit vessel can the term "recanalization" be applied if flow is restored. In the absence of knowledge of the status of the culprit vessel prior to treatment, the only fact that can be stated with certainty is the patency rate of the vessel at the moment contrast is injected. This single snapshot at a moment in time does not reflect the fluctuating status of flow in the infarct vessel that characteristically undergoes repeated cycles of patency and reocclusion, as has been documented angiographically and by continuous ST segment monitoring. Differences in efficacy between reperfusion regimens with respect to the rate and extent of improvement of flow can be discriminated better at 60 than at 90 minutes after initiation of therapy (22). Those fibrinolytic regimens that open infarct-related arteries sooner and more completely are expected to have the greatest ability to reduce infarct size and mortality.

The inadequacy of the TIMI flow grade to fully inform clinicians about the status of perfusion of the myocardium in the infarct zone led to the development of additional techniques: the TIMI frame count, TIMI myocardial perfusion grade, ST segment resolution, and myocardial contrast echocardiography (23–26). A major limitation of full-dose fibrinolytic regimens is the attainment of TIMI grade 3 flow by 60 minutes in only about 50–55% of patients, with a considerable variation in the degree of myocardial perfusion (3). The TIMI 3 flow level achieved with full-dose fibrin-specific fibrinolytics has been proposed by some investigators to be the ceiling that can be expected within the constraints of doses that can be administered safely to patients. The ability to improve myocardial perfusion is determined by multiple factors besides the flow grade in the infarct artery, such as the elapsed time from occlusion of the infarct artery, the location of the infarct artery [e.g. left anterior descending (LAD) versus non-LAD location] and the conjunctive agents administered along with the fibrinolytic (27) (Fig. 7.3).

II. ANTITHROMBINS

In the prefibrinolytic era, antithrombins were principally administered to patients with STEMI to reduce the risks of pulmonary embolism, stroke, and reinfarction. The theoretical benefits of conjunctive use of unfractionated heparin (UFH) with a fibrinolytic include the possibility of augmentation of the initial lytic effect, reduction of the risk of reocclusion of an initially successfully reperfused infarct artery (with attendant risk of reinfarction), and reduction of the risk of early mural thrombus formation (28). Despite the logic of these arguments, clinical trials of conjunctive use of UFH with fibrinolytic therapy produced confusing results that continue to impact on clinical practice. Synthesis of a large body of information on studies with UFH leads to several conclusions:

1.   Angiographic patency appears to be enhanced when UFH is administered to patients receiving a fibrin-specific fibrinolytic (29). The optimum timing of UFH relative to the fibrinolytic to achieve this goal remains uncertain, but it is common

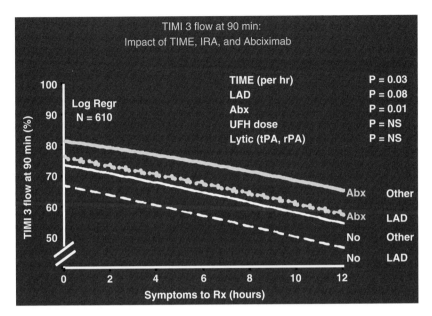

Figure 7.3 Pooled analysis of angiographic findings in alteplase and reteplase phases of TIMI 14 trial. The estimated percentage of patients achieving TIMI grade 3 flow at 90 minutes is shown versus time from onset of symptoms to initiation of the reperfusion regimen (Rx), stratified by the location of the infarct artery and whether the reperfusion regimen contained abciximab (Abx). The use of abciximab was associated with a significant increase ($p = 0.01$) in the estimated probability of achieving TIMI grade 3 flow after adjusting for time to treatment and infarct location. LAD = left anterior descending artery.

practice to administer UFH either before or shortly after (within 30–60 min) a fibrin-specific fibrinolytic has been administered (30).

2. The benefit of UFH in patients receiving streptokinase is less clear. Earlier arguments that UFH was not helpful with streptokinase may have caused clinicians to prematurely discard it as a conjunctive agent when they administered streptokinase (31). Arguments favoring the use of UFH with streptokinase include a procoagulant increase in thrombin activity after

streptokinase administration, a small reduction in mortality seen early after treatment with streptokinase, similar 5-year mortality in GUSTO I in patients who received streptokinase plus UFH versus alteplase plus UFH, and the reported beneficial effect of other antithrombins (e.g., bivalirudin, enoxaparin) on reinfarction in patients receiving streptokinase (32).

3.   Initial regimens of UFH were, in retrospect, overly aggressive and in part contributed to the risk of bleeding, especially ICH. Contemporary recommendations for use of UFH call for a weight-adjusted scheme (bolus of 60 U/kg and initial infusion of 12 U/kg/h), caps on the dose (maximum bolus 4000 U; maximum initial infusion 1000 U/h), and a target aPTT range of 1.5–2.0 times control (approximately 50–70 s) (30). Early (3-h) monitoring of the aPTT with only downward adjustment of the UFH infusion permitted at that time is helpful in reducing bleeding (17,33).

4.   When the pharmacological reperfusion regimen includes a glycoprotein IIb/IIIa inhibitor, the UFH regimen should consist of a lower weight-adjusted bolus of 40–60 U/kg followed by a reduced infusion dose of 7 U/kg/h (34,35). Selecting a bolus dose that is on the lower end of the range outlined above is preferable for the elderly as well as other patients who are at an increased risk for bleeding.

The optimum duration of UFH administration remains unsettled, but most clinicians do not feel that continuation of the infusion beyond 48 hours offers any advantage for the uncomplicated STEMI patient. Concerns about the risk of rebound activation of the coagulation cascade upon discontinuation of a UFH infusion have been raised, leading to the proposal for tapering rather than abrupt discontinuation. The benefits of such an approach await further testing.

UFH has the disadvantages of a variable anticoagulant effect, sensitivity to platelet factor 4, a relative inability to inhibit clot-bound thrombin, and the potential to cause thrombocytopenia and/or heparin-induced thrombocytopenia syndrome (28). Low molecular weight heparins (LMWHs) and direct thrombin inhibitors are the antithrombins most extensively investigated in clinical trials as alternatives to UFH in STEMI (36,37).

Phase II clinical trials (including those with LMWH as ancillary therapy to fibrinolysis and those in patients not receiving fibrinolysis) provide encouraging information suggesting that LMWH may be an attractive alternative to UFH (37). In ASSENT 3, patients received TNK and either UFH for ≥48 hours (bolus 60 U/kg; initial infusion 12 U/kg/h) or enoxaparin (bolus 30 mg; subcutaneous injections 1.0 mg/kg every 12 hours) throughout the duration of the hospital stay (35). Each element of the composite endpoint of 30-day mortality, in-hospital reinfarction, or in-hospital recurrent ischemia was reduced with enoxaparin treatment at the expense of a slight, nonsignificant increase in noncerebral bleeding complications. Results from the ASSENT 3 PLUS trial underscore the need for continued evaluation of the safety of LMWH as an adjunct to fibrinolysis (38). Among 1639 patients with STEMI receiving tenecteplase and either enoxaparin or UFH in a prehospital setting, higher rates of both major bleeding (4.0% vs. 2.8%; $p = 0.18$) and intracranial hemorrhage (2.2% vs. 1.0%; $p = 0.05$) were seen in the enoxaparin group compared with the UFH group. There was a significant interaction between patient age and risk of bleeding because almost all cases of excess intracerebral hemorrhage were confined to patients older than 75 years.

ExTRACT-TIMI 25 is a 21,000-patient trial evaluating enoxaparin versus UFH in STEMI patients receiving fibrinolytic therapy (Fig. 7.4) (38a). Importantly, it will provide information on the efficacy and safety of reduced doses of enoxaparin in the elderly. Patients in ExTRACT-TIMI 25 may be treated with approved regimens of streptokinase, t-PA, reteplase (r-PA), or TNK within 6 hours of the onset of symptoms. They are randomized to either standard weight-adjusted therapy with UFH [bolus 60 U/kg (maximum 4000 U) followed by an initial infusion of 12 U/kg/h (maximum 1000 U/h)] for at least 48 hours or to enoxaparin. For patients under 75 years, the enoxaparin regimen consists of an intravenous bolus of 30 mg followed by subcutaneous injections of 1.0 mg/kg every 12 hours. Patients 75 years or older do not receive the initial intravenous bolus and receive only 75% of the maintenance subcutaneous doses (0.75 mg/kg every 12 hours). Treatment with enoxaparin continues until hospital discharge or day 8,

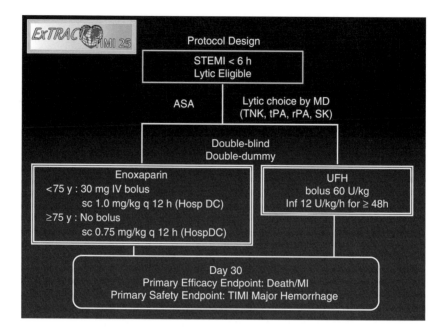

Figure 7.4 Design of ExTRACT-TIMI 25 trial. Patients with STEMI are treated with one of the four standard fibrinolytics and are randomized to receive either unfractionated heparin (UFH) or enoxaparin. Elderly patients do not receive the bolus of enoxaparin and are given only 75% of the subcutaneous dose of the younger patients.

whichever comes first. The primary endpoint is the composite of death or nonfatal reinfarction through 30 days. It is anticipated that the results of this trial will be reported in 2005.

Because clot-bound thrombin is less effectively inhibited by UFH (attachment of fibrin to the fibrin-binding domain makes the heparin-binding domain inaccessible), it was proposed that the direct antithrombins had an advantage over UFH in STEMI patients treated with a fibrinolytic because of their greater ability to block both fluid-phase and clotbound thrombin. This "thrombin hypothesis" was the basis for several randomized trials. After the TIMI 9A, GUSTO IIa, and HIT 3 trials that tested hirudin as an adjunct to fibrinolytic therapy were terminated prematurely because of excessive bleeding, the doses of both hirudin and UFH were reduced and the TIMI 9B, GUSTO IIb, and HIT 4 trials were undertaken (28). Pooled data from GUSTO IIb and TIMI 9B showed that hirudin was more effective at achieving and maintaining the target aPTT range than was UFH (28). By careful adjustment of the dose of both hirudin and UFH, major bleeding could be reduced. There was, however, no difference in mortality in UFH- vs. hirudin-treated patients; yet there was a 14% reduction in reinfarction by 30 days in patients treated with hirudin.

Possible explanations for the lack of significant benefit of hirudin in the trials noted above are:

1. Because hirudin does not block proximal portions of the coagulation cascade, once the thrombin inhibitory capacity of hirudin is exceeded, rethrombosis may occur (28).
2. Hirudin's ability to inhibit clot-bound thrombin is only about 50% of its ability to inhibit fluid-phase thrombin, reducing its potential advantage over UFH (28).
3. It is potentially possible to exhaust the available supply of hirudin in the local environment of a thrombus, thus permitting thrombin molecules to remain enzymatically active.

The HERO-2 trial evaluated the efficacy of another direct thrombin inhibitor, bivalirudin, versus UFH in conjunction with streptokinase (39). Bivalirudin did not reduce mortality compared with UFH but was associated with a lower rate of recurrent MI within 96 hours (1.6% vs. 2.3%; $p = 0.005$). Severe bleeding occurred in 0.7% of the bivalirudin group versus 0.5% for heparin ($p = 0.07$), and intracerebral bleeding occurred in 0.6% versus 0.4% ($p = 0.09$), respectively, possibly related to higher aPPT levels in the bivalirudin group. The frequency of moderate and mild bleeding was also greater with bivalirudin.

While not appearing to enhance early angiography patency compared to UFH, antithrombin alternatives to UFH studied to date do offer several advantages that make them attractive candidates for the concept of pharmacoinvasive therapy. There is a generally consistent theme of a lower rate of reocclusion of the infarct artery, reinfarction, or recurrent ischemic events. By reducing the risk of recurrent occlusion of the infarct artery and the rate of reinfarction, use of newer antithrombins would be expected to reduce the need for urgent PCI and permit consolidation of the initial benefits of pharmacological reperfusion by PCI in a more elective fashion.

Less well developed but of considerable interest are antithrombins that block even more proximally in the coagulation cascade. Given the multiplier effect of the sequence of coagulation reactions, quenching reactions proximal in the cascade has the potential to markedly decrease the amount of thrombin that is formed downstream. A phase 2 angiographic trial (PENTALYSE) evaluated fundaparinux, a synthetic pentasaccharide that is a highly selective inhibitor of factor Xa (40). The percentage of patients achieving TIMI grade 3 flow at 90 minutes was 68% in the UFH control group and ranged between 60 and 69% with low, medium, and high doses of fundaparinux. Thus, selective factor Xa inhibition may be useful in patients with STEMI and will be investigated in future phase 3 trials. Additional agents that block even more proximally to factor Xa under investigation in patients presenting with unstable angina/non ST elevation MI are the tissue factor inhibitors rNAPc2 and ch36 (41,42). Their use in STEMI has not been investigated to date.

III. ANTIPLATELET AGENTS

Platelets play a major role in the thrombotic response to rupture of a vulnerable or high-risk coronary plaque (43). Platelets are also activated in response to fibrinolysis. Based on a robust body of evidence favoring the use of aspirin in patients with a variety of vascular disorders and the 23% relative reduction in mortality with aspirin in ISIS-2, contemporary treatment regimens for STEMI include aspirin (initial dose of 162–325 mg chewed followed by maintenance dosing of 75–162 mg/d indefinitely) (44). A meta-analysis suggested that maintenance dosing with aspirin after STEMI is associated with a reduction in the risk of reinfarction (45). Thus, aspirin, one of the best studied medications in cardiovascular disease, is a key element in the pharmacotherapy of STEMI. Identification of safe and effective alternatives to aspirin is a priority in clinical trials of STEMI given the existence of patients who are allergic to aspirin and reports of patients who are resistant to its antiplatelet effects (46).

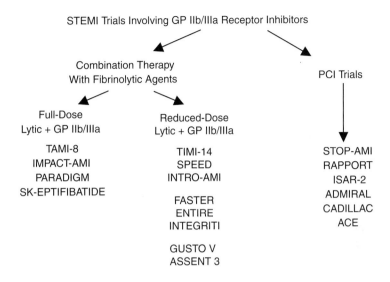

Figure 7.5 Major trials of glycoprotein IIb/IIIa inhibitors and fibrinolytics for STEMI. Pharmacological reperfusion trials are shown on the left (with full-dose fibrinolytic and reduced-dose fibrinolytic), and catheter-based reperfusion trials are shown on the right.

Irrespective of the stimulus for platelet activation, the final common pathway is expression of the activated form of the glycoprotein IIb/IIIa receptor on the platelet surface. Driven by evidence in trials of PCI that inhibitors of the glycoprotein IIb/IIIa receptor reduce the rate of ischemic events, such agents were studied in STEMI patients. Initial trials involved full-dose fibrinolytics and full-dose glycoprotein IIb/IIIa inhibitors (47–49) (Fig. 7.5). Although these studies provided proof of the concept that fibrinolytic efficacy could be enhanced by more potent antiplatelet therapy, they were associated with high rates of bleeding and alternative dosing regimens were explored (50). The majority of the data on combination reperfusion pharmacotherapy involve half the usual dose of fibrinolytics combined with a full dose of a glycoprotein IIb/IIIa inhibitor (22,51–54) (Fig. 7.5).

Pooled angiographic data from trials of combination reperfusion therapy show similar rates of TIMI 3 flow (approximately 55%) at 60

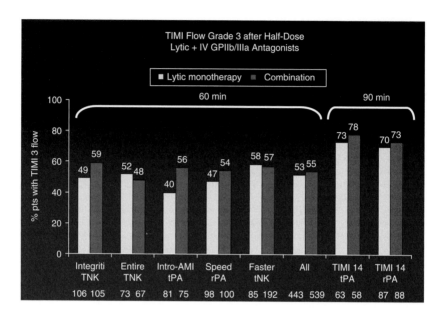

Figure 7.6   TIMI flow grade 3 at 60 and 90 minutes after initiation of fibrinolytic monotherapy and various combination reperfustion regimens for STEMI.

minutes with fibrinolytic monotherapy and combination reperfusion regimens (55) (Fig. 7.6). This finding emphasizes the central role of antiplatelet therapy in reperfusion regimens. Only half the standard dose of a fibrinolytic was used, but when complemented by conjunctive glycoprotein IIb/IIIa inhibition, the effects on the epicardial coronary artery were similar to those achieved with a full dose of the lytic agent. A number of reports involving angiographic observations and comparisons of ST segment resolution suggest that myocardial perfusion is enhanced with combination reperfusion (56,57).

    GUSTO V tested half-dose reteplase (5U and 5U) and full-dose abciximab compared with full-dose reteplase (10U and 10U) in 16,588 patients in the first 6 hours of STEMI (34). Mortality at 30 days and 1 year was similar in the full-dose reteplase and combination reperfusion groups. However, nonfatal reinfarction and other complications of MI were reduced in the combination reperfusion therapy group. Although the rates of ICH were the same in the two treatment groups (0.6%), moderate to severe bleeding was significantly increased from 2.3 to 4.6% with combination reperfusion therapy ($p < 0.001$). This excess bleeding risk appeared to be limited to those over the age of 75 years. Similar to the GUSTO V trial, combination reperfusion therapy with half-dose tenecteplase and abciximab in the ASSENT 3 trial was not associated with a reduction in 30-day mortality (35). In-hospital reinfarction and refractory ischemia were reduced with combination reperfusion therapy, but this occurred at the expense of an increase in major bleeding other than ICH. The elderly were at greatest risk for excess bleeding, experiencing a threefold increase in the rate of this complication.

The failure of combination reperfusion pharmacotherapy to translate into a mortality benefit in either the short or the long term was a disappointment that dampened initial enthusiasm for its becoming a replacement for full-dose fibrinolysis (58). Potential explanations for the observations to date include:

1. Lack of a major difference in early TIMI 3 flow rates produced little difference in myocardial salvage.
2. The magnitude of the difference in reinfarction was too small to impact on mortality
3. The increased bleeding, especially fatal ICHs in the elderly, may have offset any mortality advantage associated with better myocardial perfusion.
4. The beneficial effects of other contemporary therapies such as aspirin, beta-blockers, and inhibitors of the renin-angiotensin-aldosterone system as well as an aggressive approach to revascularization following STEMI may override any small differences in myocardial perfusion related to the acute reperfusion therapy administered.

Intravenous glycoprotein IIb/IIIa inhibitors have also been evaluated in patients undergoing primary PCI. The STOPAMI trial showed improved myocardial salvage when abciximab was combined with coronary stenting versus pharamcologic reperfusion with t-PA (59). Clinical endpoints were reported in the RAPPORT, ISAR-2, ADMI-RAL, CADILLAC, and ACE trials in which abciximab was compared to placebo in patients undergoing primary PCI (60). In the collective dataset of these five trials, 3666 patients were randomized, half of whom received abciximab. This limited sample size coupled with the difficulty of diagnosing periprocedural MI in patients undergoing PCI for STEMI limits the ability to draw definitive conclusions about the role of abciximab. Assessment of the impact of abciximab varies depending on the definition of the composite endpoint in the trial — endpoints of death/MI or death/MI/urgent TVR showed benefit of abciximab with most of the protective effect coming from a reduction of recurrent infarction or urgent TVR.

It cannot be stated with certainty that all patients who undergo primary PCI with stenting benefit from abciximab. The CADILLAC trial enrolled a relatively low-risk population of patients and failed to show an incremental advantage of abciximab plus stenting versus stenting alone (61). In contrast, in patients presenting with cardiogenic shock, treatment with abciximab is associated with especially large treatment benefits on mortality, reinfarction, and urgent target vessel revascularization (62–65). The magnitude of the treatment effect of abciximab in cardiogenic shock may be related to the particularly adverse impact of microvascular obstruction in the presence of severely compromised myocardial function and the beneficial effects of abciximab on such obstructions.

Only a modest amount of angiographic data are available on the small molecular glycoprotein IIb/IIIa inhibitors in STEMI (66). However, based on a common mechanism of action, tirofiban or eptifibatide may also be useful as antiplatelet therapy to support primary PCI for STEMI.

Substantial evidence supports the use of the thienopyridine clopidogrel in patients with UA/NSTEMI who are treated medically or who undergo PCI with stenting (67,68). Clopidogrel is also used, in combination with aspirin, following elective PCI with stenting (69). Information on the efficacy and safety of dual antiplatelet therapy with

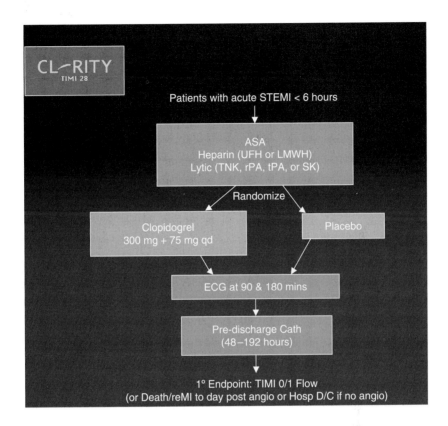

Figure 7.7 Design of CLARITY-TIMI 28 trial.

aspirin and clopidogrel in STEMI patients will be forthcoming from several ongoing trials. CLARITY-TIMI 28 is studying the impact of combination of aspirin plus clopidogrel versus aspirin alone on angiographic patency of the infarct artery in patients with STEMI who receive a fibrinolytic (Fig. 7.7). COMMIT is studying aspirin plus clopidogrel versus aspirin alone with respect to mortality and the composite of death/MI/CVA in patients presenting with a suspected MI within the preceding 24 hours; a large proportion of the patients in COMMIT will be STEMI patients who receive a fibrinolytic (Fig. 7.8).

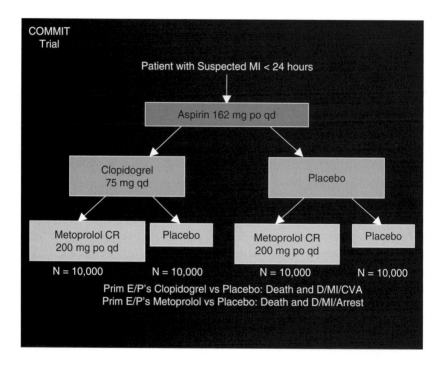

Figure 7.8 Design of COMMIT trial.

IV. ADJUNCTIVE AGENTS FOR MYOCARDIAL PROTECTION

Agents investigated for protection of the infarcting myocardium may be broadly grouped into three partially overlapping categories of those that (a) improve the integrity and function of the microvasculature, (b) prevent inflammatory damage, and (c) provide metabolic support for the infarcting myocardium (Fig. 7.9).

The antithrombins and antiplatelet agents discussed above are examples of interventions that protect the integrity of the microvasculature in the infarct zone (27,70). However, any agent that decreases inflammation and myocyte swelling also protects the microvasculature. Specific anti-inflammatory interventions that have been tested in contemporary STEMI

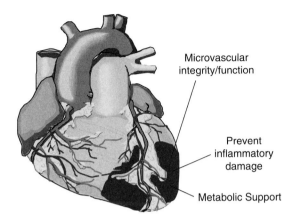

Microvascular
integrity/function

Prevent
inflammatory
damage

Metabolic Support

Figure 7.9　Major categories of myocardial protection therapies for STEMI.

trials include anti-adhesion (antiCD18), anti-P-selectin, and anticomplement molecules (71–75). Although each of these categories of anti-inflammatory molecules showed promise in animal models, they failed to reduce infarct size when evaluated in clinical trials. With the exception of pexelizumab, a monoclonal antibody against the C5 component complement, the lack of benefit in phase 2 clinical trials halted further development. In the COMMA trial, pexelizumab treatment during angioplasty significantly reduced mortality at 90 days compared with placebo (1.8% vs. 5.9%; $p = 0.014$). This served as the foundation for a phase III trial of pexelizumab (75).

A large array of agents has been tested for metabolic protection of the myocardium, but most have been discarded either after proving ineffective in clinical trials or protective in only a limited subset of STEMI patients. Some interest in glucose-insulin-potassium (GIK) continues to exist, but it is likely that the volume load associated with its administration will limit GIK to patients without significant pump dysfunction (76).

Several issues are worthy of consideration when interpreting randomized trials of anti-inflammatory treatments and metabolic support for STEMI. A consistent pattern of a sound biological hypothesis and promising animal models is typically followed by disappointing results in phase II trials. This raises the question as to whether animal models accurately predict clinical outcomes in patients with STEMI. Investigators can control with great precision the timing and extent of myocardial damage in animal models. Such models, which characteristically utilize a ligature or snare on the target coronary artery, may not reflect the more diffuse nature of atherosclerosis in patients where multiple zones of ischemia and fluctuating collateral flow may be operative. In addition, it appears important to have the myocardial protective agent in place at the time coronary occlusion occurs — something easily accomplished in animal models but almost impossible clinically. Administration of the agent at the time of initiation of reperfusion or late after reperfusion has begun is unlikely to have a significant impact on myocardial salvage. Phase II trials of new myocardial protective agents typically proceed cautiously and focus on selected groups of patients, often eliminating those with cardiogenic shock. Finally, given the marked improvements in mortality and morbidity associated with early reperfusion, aspirin, beta blockade, and inhibition of the renin angiotensin aldosterone system in contemporary management of STEMI, it is increasingly difficult to detect a signal of incremental benefit from a myocardial protective agent.

One potential therapy that may circumvent the deficiencies described above is inhibition of caspases responsible for apoptosis of myocytes (77). Apoptosis, a more slowly developing process after STEMI that results in the dropout of myocytes, may still be amenable to pharmacological maneuvers even after reperfusion has occurred.

V. THE FUTURE OF PHARMACOINVASIVE THERAPY

Identification of optimal care for the patient with STEMI is challenging because of the dynamic nature of the evidence base on which clinical decisions are made. The introduction of new agents and devices and refinement of treatment strategies rapidly make prior studies less relevant to contemporary practice. An example of this concept is the prior proscription against routine catheterization and intervention within the first 24 hours after fibrinolysis (78–80). Such an admonition, correct at the time it was made more than a decade ago, is almost certainly not so today. Improvements in imaging equipment, guidewires, catheters, antithrombotic support at the time of PCI, and availability of stents, embolectomy devices, distal protection devices, and circulatory support devices have improved the safety and efficacy of early PCI after fibrinolysis. Creating a mindset in which routine PCI after fibrinolysis is no longer proscribed but is encouraged captures the advantage of earlier initiation of reperfusion therapy beginning with a pharmacological approach followed by several additional benefits provided in the catheterization laboratory: enhancement of flow in the epicardial infarct artery through balloon dilation and stenting, improved myocardial perfusion, and consolidation of the initial benefits of pharmacological reperfusion by minimizing the risk of recurrent infarction and ischemia.

Movement toward a pharmacoinvasive approach requires data from randomized trials to provide the necessary evidence to shift medical practice. It is likely that in the future the initial pharmacological reperfusion administered will need to be customized based on the risk of the STEMI and the risk of bleeding. Potential regimens, to be followed by early PCI, include:

1. Combination reperfusion therapy with reduced-dose fibrinolytic and a glycoprotein IIb/IIIa inhibitor for patients with a large quantity of anterior myocardium at risk and at low risk for bleeding.
2. Full-dose fibrinolysis without a glycoprotein IIb/IIIa inhibitor but with a conservative dosing scheme of an antithrombin in patients at increased risk of bleeding. The full dose of a fibrinolytic in those above the age of 75 will likely need to be reduced, perhaps by as much as 25%.
3. Glycoprotein IIb/IIIa inhibitor therapy alone for patients at the highest risk of bleeding.

We believe that it is only a matter of time before UFH is replaced by one of the antithrombins currently being studied. At present, most of the evidence suggests that in the near future it is likely to be enoxaparin. Reduction of the dose of enoxaparin in the elderly hopefully will reduce the risk of bleeding (Fig. 7.4). Further measures that appear promising are bedside assays to provide a guide to the levels of anti-Xa activity (81). Valuable information to address these areas will be forthcoming from the ongoing ASSENT 4 PCI and FINESSE studies.

The role of thienopyridines in patients receiving fibrinolytics remains uncertain. Issues of when to administer a thienopyridine relative to the fibrinolytic and whether a loading dose is effective and safe require clarification (Fig. 7.7).

Finally, although there continues to be a sound biological rationale for administering a myocardial protective agent as part of the reperfusion strategy, we remain concerned about the ability to deliver such therapies early enough in the evolving infarction process. Myocardial protective therapies that have less time dependency relative to coronary occlusion and reperfusion have the greatest potential for being added to future STEMI regimens.

REFERENCES

1. Schomig A, Ndrepepa G, Mehilli J, Schwaiger M, Schuhlen H, Nekolla S, Pache J, Martinoff S, Bollwein H, Kastrati A. Therapy-dependent influence of time-to-treatment interval on myocardial salvage in patients with acute myocardial infarction treated with coronary artery stenting or thrombolysis. Circulation. 2003;108:1084–1088.

2. Gibson CM. Time is myocardium and time is outcomes. Circulation. 2001;104:2632–2634.

3. Waters RE II, Mahaffey KW, Granger CB, Roe MT. Current perspectives on reperfusion therapy for acute ST-segment elevation myocardial infarction: integrating pharmacologic and mechanical reperfusion strategies. Am Heart J. 2003;146:958–968.

4. Katritsis D, Karvouni E, Webb-Peploe MM. Reperfusion in acute myocardial infarction: current concepts. Prog Cardiovasc Dis. 2003;45:481–492.

5. Dauerman HL, Sobel BE. Synergistic treatment of ST-segment elevation myocardial infarction with pharmacoinvasive recanalization. J Am Coll Cardiol. 2003;42:646–51.

6. TIMI Study Group. The Thrombolysis in Myocardial Infarction (TIMI) trial. Phase I findings. N Engl J Med. 1985;312:932–936.

7. The GUSTO Investigators. An international randomized trial comparing four thrombolytic strategies for acute myocardial infarction. N Engl J Med. 1993;329:673–682.

8. The GUSTO Angiographic Investigators. The comparative effects of tissue plasminogen activator, streptokinase, or both on coronary artery patency, ventricular function and survival after acute myocardial infarction. N Engl J Med. 1993;329:1615–1622.

9. Llevadot J, Giugliano RP, Antman EM. Bolus fibrinolytic therapy in acute myocardial infarction. JAMA. 2001;286:442–449.

10. The Global Use of Strategies to Open Occluded Coronary Arteries (GUSTO III) Investigators. A comparison of reteplase with alteplase for acute myocardial infarction. N Engl J Med. 1997;337:1118–1123.

11. Assessment of the Safety and Efficacy of a New Thrombolytic (ASSENT 2) Investigators. Single-bolus tenecteplase compared with front-loaded alteplase in acute myocardial infarction: the ASSENT-2 double-blind randomised trial. Lancet. 1999;354:716–722.

12. The InTIME-II Investigators. Intravenous NPA for the treatment of infarcting myocardium early; InTIME-II, a double-blind comparison of single-bolus lanoteplase vs. accelerated alteplase for the treatment of patients with acute myocardial infarction. Eur Heart J. 2000;21: 2005–2013.

13. Ware JH, Antman EM. Equivalence trials. N Engl J Med. 1997;337: 1159–1161.

14. Cannon CP, McCabe CH, Gibson CM, Ghali M, Sequeira RF, McKendall GR, Breed J, Modi NB, Fox NL, Tracy RP, Love TW, Braunwald E. TNK-tissue plasminogen activator in acute myocardial infarction. Results of the Thrombolysis in Myocardial Infarction (TIMI) 10A dose-ranging trial. Circulation. 1997;95:351–356.

15. Cannon CP, Gibson CM, McCabe CH, Adgey AA, Schweiger MJ, Sequeira RF, Grollier G, Giugliano RP, Frey M, Mueller HS, Steingart RM, Weaver WD, Van de Werf F, Braunwald E. TNK-tissue plasminogen activator compared with front-loaded alteplase in acute myocardial infarction: results of the TIMI 10B trial. Thrombolysis in Myocardial Infarction (TIMI) 10B Investigators. Circulation. 1998;98: 2805–2814.

16. Van de Werf F, Cannon CP, Luyten A, Houbracken K, McCabe CH, Berioli S, Bluhmki E, Sarelin H, Wang-Clow F, Fox NL, Braunwald E. Safety assessment of single-bolus administration of TNK tissue-plasminogen activator in acute myocardial infarction: the ASSENT-1 trial. The ASSENT-1 Investigators. Am Heart J. 1999;137:786–791.

17. Giugliano RP, McCabe CH, Antman EM, Cannon CP, Van de Werf F, Wilcox RG, Braunwald E. Lower-dose heparin with fibrinolysis is associated with lower rates of intracranial hemorrhage. Am Heart J. 2001;141:742–750.

18. Fibrinolytic Therapy Trialists' (FTT) Collaborative Group. Indications for fibrinolytic therapy in suspected acute myocardial infarction: collaborative overview of early mortality and major morbidity results from all randomised trials of more than 1000 patients. Lancet. 1994;343: 311–322.

19. Gore JM, Granger CB, Simoons ML, Sloan MA, Weaver WD, White HD, Barbash GI, Van de Werf F, Aylward PE, Topol EJ, et al. Stroke after thrombolysis. Mortality and functional outcomes in the GUSTO-I trial. Global Use of Strategies To Open Occluded Coronary Arteries. Circulation. 1995;92:2811–2818.

20. Simoons ML, Maggioni AP, Knatterud G, Leimberger JD, de Jaegere P, van Domburg R, Boersma E, Franzosi MG, Califf R, Schroder R, et al. Individual risk assessment for intracranial haemorrhage during thrombolytic therapy. Lancet. 1993;342:1523–1528.

21. Chesebro JH, Knatterud G, Roberts R, Borer J, Cohen LS, Dalen J, Dodge HT, Francis CK, Hillis D, Ludbrook P, et al. Thrombolysis in Myocardial Infarction (TIMI) Trial, Phase I: A comparison between intravenous tissue plasminogen activator and intravenous streptokinase. Clinical findings through hospital discharge. Circulation. 1987;76: 142–154.

22. Antman EM, Giugliano RP, Gibson CM, McCabe CH, Coussement P, Kleiman NS, Vahanian A, Adgey AA, Menown I, Rupprecht HJ, Van der Wieken R, Ducas J, Scherer J, Anderson K, Van de Werf F, Braunwald E. Abciximab facilitates the rate and extent of thrombolysis: results of the thrombolysis in myocardial infarction (TIMI) 14 trial. The TIMI 14 Investigators. Circulation. 1999;99:2720–2732.

23. Gibson CM, Murphy SA, Rizzo MJ, Ryan KA, Marble SJ, McCabe CH, Cannon CP, Van de Werf F, Braunwald E. Relationship between TIMI frame count and clinical outcomes after thrombolytic administration. Thrombolysis In Myocardial Infarction (TIMI) Study Group. Circulation. 1999;99:1945–1950.

24. Gibson CM, Cannon CP, Murphy SA, Ryan KA, Mesley R, Marble SJ, McCabe CH, Van De Werf F, Braunwald E. Relationship of TIMI myocardial perfusion grade to mortality after administration of thrombolytic drugs. Circulation. 2000;101:125–130.

25. Angeja BG, Gunda M, Murphy SA, Sobel BE, Rundle AC, Syed M, Asfour A, Borzak S, Gourlay SG, Barron HV, Gibbons RJ, Gibson CM. TIMI myocardial perfusion grade and ST segment resolution: association with infarct size as assessed by single photon emission computed tomography imaging. Circulation. 2002;105:282–285.

26. Armstrong PW, Collen D, Antman E. Fibrinolysis for acute myocardial infarction: the future is here and now. Circulation. 2003;107:2533–2537.

27. Antman EM, Cooper HA, Gibson CM, de Lemos JA, McCabe CH, Giugliano RP, Coussement P, Murphy S, Scherer J, Anderson K, Van de Werf F, Braunwald E. Determinants of improvement in epicardial flow and myocardial perfusion for ST elevation myocardial infarction; insights from TIMI 14 and InTIME-II. Eur Heart J. 2002;23:928–933.

28. Antman EM. The search for replacements for unfractionated heparin. Circulation. 2001;103:2310–2314.

29. Mahaffey KW, Granger CB, Collins R, O'Connor CM, Ohman EM, Bleich SD, Col JJ, Califf RM. Overview of randomized trials of intravenous heparin in patients with acute myocardial infarction treated with thrombolytic therapy. Am J Cardiol. 1996;77:551–556.

30. Menon V, Berkowitz SD, Antman EM, Fuchs RM, Hochman JS. New heparin dosing recommendations for patients with acute coronary syndromes. Am J Med. 2001;110:641–650.

31. Collins R, Peto R, Baigent C, Sleight P. Aspirin, heparin, and fibrinolytic therapy in suspected acute myocardial infarction. N Engl J Med. 1997;336:847–860.

32. White H. Further evidence that antithrombotic therapy is beneficial with streptokinase: improved early ST resolution and late patency with enoxaparin. Eur Heart J. 2002;23:1233–1237.

33. Giugliano RP, Antman EM. Caeteris paribus — all things being equal. Eur Heart J. 2001;22:2221–2223.

34. Topol EJ. Reperfusion therapy for acute myocardial infarction with fibrinolytic therapy or combination reduced fibrinolytic therapy and platelet glycoprotein IIb/IIIa inhibition: the GUSTO V randomised trial. Lancet. 2001;357:1905–1914.

35. Assessment of the Safety and Efficacy of a New Thrombolytic (ASSENT 3) Investigators. Efficacy and safety of tenecteplase in combination with enoxaparin, abciximab, or unfractionated heparin: the ASSENT-3 randomised trial in acute myocardial infarction. Lancet. 2001;358:605–613.

36. The Direct Thrombin Inhibitor Trialists' Collaborative Group. Direct thrombin inhibitors in acute coronary syndromes: principal results of a meta-analysis based on individual patients' data. Lancet. 2002;359:294–302.

37. Wong GC, Giugliano RP, Antman EM. Use of low-molecular-weight heparins in the management of acute coronary artery syndromes and percutaneous coronary intervention. JAMA. 2003;289:331–342.

38. Wallentin L, Goldstein P, Armstrong PW, Granger CB, Adgey AA, Arntz HR, Bogaerts K, Danays T, Lindahl B, Makijarvi M, Verheugt F, Van de Werf F. Efficacy and safety of tenecteplase in combination with the low-molecular-weight heparin enoxaparin or unfractionated heparin in the prehospital setting: the Assessment of the Safety and Efficacy of a New Thrombolytic Regimen (ASSENT)-3 PLUS randomized trial in acute myocardial infarction. Circulation. 2003;108:135–142.

38a. Antman EM, Morrow DA, McCabe CH, Jiang F, White HD, Fox KAA, Chew P, Braunwald E, for the ExTRACT-TIMI 25 Investigators. Enoxaparin versus unfractionated heparin as antithrombin therapy in patients receiving fibrinolysis for ST elevation MI: Design and rationale for the EnoXaparin and Thrombolysis Reperfusion for Acute myocardial infarCtion Treatment Thrombolysis in Myocardial Infarction-Study 25 (ExTRACT-TIMI 25). American Heart J. In press.

39. White H. Thrombin-specific anticoagulation with bivalirudin versus heparin in patients receiving fibrinolytic therapy for acute myocardial infarction: the HERO-2 randomised trial. Lancet. 2001;358:1855–1863.

40. Coussement PK, Bassand JP, Convens C, Vrolix M, Boland J, Grollier G, Michels R, Vahanian A, Vanderheyden M, Rupprecht HJ, Van de Werf F. A synthetic factor-Xa inhibitor (ORG31540/SR9017A) as an adjunct to fibrinolysis in acute myocardial infarction. The PENTAL-YSE study. Eur Heart J. 2001;22:1716–1724.

41. Moons AH, Peters RJ, Bijsterveld NR, Piek JJ, Prins MH, Vlasuk GP, Rote WE, Buller HR. Recombinant nematode anticoagulant protein c2, an inhibitor of the tissue factor/factor VIIa complex, in patients undergoing elective coronary angioplasty. J Am Coll Cardiol. 2003;41: 2147–2153.

42. Nylander S, Mattsson C. Thrombin-induced platelet activation and its inhibition by anticoagulants with different modes of action. Blood Coagul Fibrinolysis. 2003;14:159–167.

43. Naghavi M, Libby P, Falk E, Casscells SW, Litovsky S, Rumberger J, Badimon JJ, Stefanadis C, Moreno P, Pasterkamp G, Fayad Z, Stone PH, Waxman S, Raggi P, Madjid M, Zarrabi A, Burke A, Yuan C, Fitzgerald PJ, Siscovick DS, de Korte CL, Aikawa M, Juhani Airaksinen KE, Assmann G, Becker CR, Chesebro JH, Farb A, Galis ZS, Jackson C, Jang IK, Koenig W, Lodder RA, March K, Demirovic J, Navab M, Priori SG, Rekhter MD, Bahr R, Grundy SM, Mehran R, Colombo A, Boerwinkle E, Ballantyne C, Insull W, Jr., Schwartz RS, Vogel R, Serruys PW, Hansson GK, Faxon DP, Kaul S, Drexler H, Greenland P, Muller JE, Virmani R, Ridker PM, Zipes DP, Shah PK, Willerson JT. From vulnerable plaque to vulnerable patient: a call for new definitions and risk assessment strategies: Part I. Circulation. 2003;108:1664–1672.

44. ISIS-2 (Second International Study of Infarct Survival) Collaborative Group. Randomised trial of intravenous streptokinase, oral aspirin, both, or neither among 17,187 cases of suspected acute myocardial infarction: ISIS-2. Lancet. 1988;2:349–360.

45. Roux S, Christeller S, Ludin E. Effects of aspirin on coronary reocclusion and recurrent ischemia after thrombolysis: a meta-analysis. J Am Coll Cardiol. 1992;19:671–677.

46. Schafer AI. Genetic and acquired determinants of individual variability of response to antiplatelet drugs. Circulation. 2003;108:910–911.

47. Kleiman NS, Ohman EM, Califf RM, George BS, Kereiakes D, Aguirre FV, Weisman H, Schaible T, Topol EJ. Profound inhibition of platelet aggregation with monoclonal antibody 7E3 Fab after thrombolytic therapy. Results of the Thrombolysis and Angioplasty in Myocardial Infarction (TAMI) 8 Pilot Study. J Am Coll Cardiol. 1993;22:381–389.

48. Ohman EM, Kleiman NS, Gacioch G, Worley SJ, Navetta FI, Talley JD, Anderson HV, Ellis SG, Cohen MD, Spriggs D, Miller M, Kere-iakes D, Yakubov S, Kitt MM, Sigmon KN, Califf RM, Krucoff MW, Topol EJ. Combined accelerated tissue-plasminogen activator and platelet glycoprotein IIb/IIIa integrin receptor blockade with Integrilin in acute myocardial infarction. Results of a randomized, placebo-con-trolled, dose-ranging trial. IMPACT-AMI Investigators. Circulation. 1997;95:846–854.

49. The PARADIGM Investigators. Combining thrombolysis with the platelet glycoprotein IIb/IIIa inhibitor lamifiban: results of the Platelet Aggregation Receptor Antagonist Dose Investigation and Reperfusion Gain in Myocardial Infarction (PARADIGM) trial. J Am Coll Cardiol. 1998;32:2003–2010.

50. Ronner E, van Kesteren HA, Zijnen P, Altmann E, Molhoek PG, van der Wieken LR, Cuffie-Jackson CA, Neuhaus KL, Simoons ML. Safety and efficacy of eptifibatide vs. placebo in patients receiving throm-bolytic therapy with streptokinase for acute myocardial infarction; a phase II dose escalation, randomized, double-blind study. Eur Heart J. 2000;21:1530–1536.

51. Antman EM, Gibson CM, de Lemos JA, Giugliano RP, McCabe CH, Coussement P, Menown I, Nienaber CA, Rehders TC, Frey MJ, Van der Wieken R, Andresen D, Scherer J, Anderson K, Van de Werf F, Braunwald E. Combination reperfusion therapy with abciximab and reduced dose reteplase: results from TIMI 14. The Thrombolysis in Myocardial Infarc-tion (TIMI) 14 Investigators. Eur Heart J. 2000;21: 1944–1953.

52. Brener SJ, Zeymer U, Adgey AA, Vrobel TR, Ellis SG, Neuhaus KL, Juran N, Ivanc TB, Ohman EM, Strony J, Kitt M, Topol EJ. Eptifibatide and low-dose tissue plasminogen activator in acute myocardial infarc-tion: the Integrilin and Low-Dose Thrombolysis in Acute Myocardial Infarction (INTRO AMI) trial. J Am Coll Cardiol. 2002;39:377–386.

53. Strategies for Patency Enhancement in the Emergency Department (SPEED) Group. Trial of abciximab with and without low-dose reteplase for acute myocardial infarction. Circulation. 2000;101:2788– 2794.

54. Giugliano RP, Roe MT, Harrington RA, Gibson CM, Zeymer U, Van de Werf F, Baran KW, Hobbach HP, Woodlief LH, Hannan KL, Greenberg S, Miller J, Kitt MM, Strony J, McCabe CH, Braunwald E, Califf RM. Combination reperfusion therapy with eptifibatide and reduced-dose tenecteplase for ST-elevation myocardial infarction: results of the Integrilin and Tenecteplase in Acute Myocardial Infarction (INTEGRITI) Phase II Angiographic Trial. J Am Coll Cardiol. 2003;41:1251– 1260.

55. Ohman EM, Oliverio RM, Harrelson L. Results of the Fibrinolytics and Aggrastat in ST Elevation Resolution (FASTER, TIMI 24) randomized trial. In press. 2004.

56. de Lemos JA, Antman EM, Gibson CM, McCabe CH, Giugliano RP, Murphy SA, Coulter SA, Anderson K, Scherer J, Frey MJ, Van Der Wieken R, Van De Werf F, Braunwald E. Abciximab improves both epicardial flow and myocardial reperfusion in ST-elevation myocardial infarction. Observations from the TIMI 14 trial. Circulation. 2000;101: 239–243.

57. Gibson CM, de Lemos JA, Murphy SA, Marble SJ, McCabe CH, Cannon CP, Antman EM, Braunwald E. Combination therapy with abciximab reduces angiographically evident thrombus in acute myocardial infarction: a TIMI 14 substudy. Circulation. 2001;103:2550– 2554.

58. Lincoff AM, Califf RM, Van de Werf F, Willerson JT, White HD, Armstrong PW, Guetta V, Gibler WB, Hochman JS, Bode C, Vahanian A, Steg PG, Ardissino D, Savonitto S, Bar F, Sadowski Z, Betriu A, Booth JE, Wolski K, Waller M, Topol EJ. Mortality at 1 year with combination platelet glycoprotein IIb/IIIa inhibition and reduced-dose fibrinolytic therapy vs. conventional fibrinolytic therapy for acute myocardial infarction: GUSTO V randomized trial. JAMA 2002;288:2130– 2135.

59. Schomig A, Kastrati A, Dirschinger J, Mehilli J, Schricke U, Pache J, Martinoff S, Neumann FJ, Schwaiger M. Coronary stenting plus platelet glycoprotein IIb/IIIa blockade compared with tissue plasminogen activator in acute myocardial infarction. Stent versus Thrombolysis for

Occluded Coronary Arteries in Patients with Acute Myocardial Infarction Study Investigators. N Engl J Med. 2000;343:385–391.

60. Topol EJ, Neumann FJ, Montalescot G. A preferred reperfusion strategy for acute myocardial infarction. J Am Coll Cardiol. 2003;42:1886– 1889.

61. Stone GW, Grines CL, Cox DA, Garcia E, Tcheng JE, Griffin JJ, Guagliumi G, Stuckey T, Turco M, Carroll JD, Rutherford BD, Lansky AJ. Comparison of angioplasty with stenting, with or without abciximab, in acute myocardial infarction. N Engl J Med. 2002;346:957– 966.

62. Montalescot G, Barragan P, Wittenberg O, Ecollan P, Elhadad S, Villain P, Boulenc JM, Morice MC, Maillard L, Pansieri M, Choussat R, Pinton P. Platelet glycoprotein IIb/IIIa inhibition with coronary stenting for acute myocardial infarction. N Engl J Med. 2001;344:1895–1903.

63. Giri S, Mitchel J, Azar RR, Kiernan FJ, Fram DB, McKay RG, Mennett R, Clive J, Hirst JA. Results of primary percutaneous transluminal coronary angioplasty plus abciximab with or without stenting for acute myocardial infarction complicated by cardiogenic shock. Am J Cardiol. 2002;89:126–131.

64. Chan AW, Chew DP, Bhatt DL, Moliterno DJ, Topol EJ, Ellis SG. Long-term mortality benefit with the combination of stents and abciximab for cardiogenic shock complicating acute myocardial infarction. Am J Cardiol. 2002;89:132–136.

65. Antoniucci D, Valenti R, Migliorini A, Moschi G, Trapani M, Dovellini EV, Bolognese L, Santoro GM. Abciximab therapy improves survival in patients with acute myocardial infarction complicated by early cardiogenic shock undergoing coronary artery stent implantation. Am J Cardiol. 2002;90:353–357.

66. Lee DP, Herity NA, Hiatt BL, Fearon WF, Rezaee M, Carter AJ, Huston M, Schreiber D, DiBattiste PM, Yeung AC. Adjunctive platelet glycoprotein IIb/IIIa receptor inhibition with tirofiban before primary angioplasty improves angiographic outcomes: results of the TIrofiban Given in the Emergency Room before Primary Angioplasty (TIGER-PA) pilot trial. Circulation. 2003;107:1497–1501.

67. CAPRIE Steering Committee. A randomised, blinded, trial of clopidogrel versus aspirin in patients at risk of ischaemic events (CAPRIE). Lancet. 1996;348:1329–1339.

68. Yusuf S, Zhao F, Mehta SR, Chrolavicius S, Tognoni G, Fox KK. Effects of clopidogrel in addition to aspirin in patients with acute coronary syndromes without ST-segment elevation. N Engl J Med. 2001;345:494–502.

69. Lange RA, Hillis LD. Antiplatelet therapy for ischemic heart disease. N Engl J Med. 2004;350:277–280.

70. de Lemos JA, Gibson CM, Antman EM, Murphy SA, Morrow DA, Schuhwerk KC, Schweiger M, Coussement P, Van de Werf F, Braunwald E. Abciximab and early adjunctive percutaneous coronary intervention are associated with improved ST-segment resolution after thrombolysis: Observations from the TIMI 14 trial. Am Heart J. 2001; 141:592–598.

71. Baran KW, Nguyen M, McKendall GR, Lambrew CT, Dykstra G, Palmeri ST, Gibbons RJ, Borzak S, Sobel BE, Gourlay SG, Rundle AC, Gibson CM, Barron HV. Double-blind, randomized trial of an anti-CD18 antibody in conjunction with recombinant tissue plasminogen activator for acute myocardial infarction: Limitation of Myocardial Infarction Following Thrombolysis in Acute Myocardial Infarction (LIMIT AMI) study. Circulation. 2001;104:2778–2783.

72. Faxon DP, Gibbons RJ, Chronos NA, Gurbel PA, Sheehan F. The effect of blockade of the CD11/CD18 integrin receptor on infarct size in patients with acute myocardial infarction treated with direct angioplasty: the results of the HALT-MI study. J Am Coll Cardiol. 2002;40: 1199–1204.

73. Wang K, Zhou X, Zhou Z, Tarakji K, Qin JX, Sitges M, Shiota T, Forudi F, Schaub RG, Kumar A, Penn MS, Topol EJ, Lincoff AM. Recombinant soluble P-selectin glycoprotein ligand-Ig (rPSGL-Ig) attenuates infarct size and myeloperoxidase activity in a canine model of ischemia-reperfusion. Thromb Haemost. 2002;88:149–154.

74. Mahaffey KW, Granger CB, Nicolau JC, Ruzyllo W, Weaver WD, Theroux P, Hochman JS, Filloon TG, Mojcik CF, Todaro TG, Armstrong PW. Effect of pexelizumab, an anti-C5 complement antibody, as adjunctive therapy to fibrinolysis in acute myocardial infarction: the COMPlement inhibition in myocardial infarction treated with thromboLYtics (COMPLY) trial. Circulation. 2003;108:1176–1183.

75. Granger CB, Mahaffey KW, Weaver WD, Theroux P, Hochman JS, Filloon TG, Rollins S, Todaro TG, Nicolau JC, Ruzyllo W, Armstrong PW. Pexelizumab, an anti-C5 complement antibody, as adjunctive therapy to primary percutaneous coronary intervention in acute myocardial infarction: the COMplement inhibition in Myocardial infarction treated with Angioplasty (COMMA) trial. Circulation. 2003;108:1184–1190.

76. Apstein CS. The benefits of glucose-insulin-potassium for acute myocardial infarction (and some concerns). J Am Coll Cardiol. 2003;42: 792–795.

77. Guttenplan N, Lee C, Frishman WH. Inhibition of myocardial apoptosis as a therapeutic target in cardiovascular disease prevention: focus on caspase inhibition. Heart Dis. 2001;3:313–318.

78. The TIMI Study Group. Comparison of invasive and conservative strategies after treatment with intravenous tissue plasminogen activator in acute myocardial infarction. Results of the Thrombolysis in Myocardial Infarction (TIMI) phase II trial. N Engl J Med. 1989;320: 618–627.

79. Arnold AE, Simoons ML, Van de Werf F, de Bono DP, Lubsen J, Tijssen JG, Serruys PW, Verstraete M. Recombinant tissue-type plasminogen activator and immediate angioplasty in acute myocardial infarction. One-year follow-up. The European Cooperative Study Group. Circulation. 1992;86:111–120.

80. SWIFT (Should We Intervene Following Thrombolysis?) Trial Study Group. SWIFT trial of delayed elective intervention v conservative treatment after thrombolysis with anistreplase in acute myocardial infarction. BMJ. 1991;302:555–560.

81. Moliterno DJ, Hermiller JB, Kereiakes DJ, Yow E, Applegate RJ, Braden GA, Dippel EJ, Furman MI, Grines CL, Kleiman NS, Levine GN, Mann T III, Nair RN, Stine RA, Yacubov SJ, Tcheng JE. A novel point-of-care enoxaparin monitor for use during percutaneous coronary intervention. Results of the Evaluating Enoxaparin Clotting Times (ELECT) Study. J Am Coll Cardiol. 2003;42:1132–1139.

III

Definitive Assessment of Pharmacoinvasive Therapy in the Treatment of STEMI

8

Design and Overview of Contemporary Studies of Pharmacoinvasive Therapy

KANWAR SINGH, MATTHEW ROE, and ROBERT HARRINGTON

Duke Clinical Research Institute,
Durham, North Carolina, U.S.A.

I. INTRODUCTION

The challenge facing proponents of pharmacoinvasive therapy (1) lies in translating the potential synergistic benefits of a combined pharmacological and mechanical reperfusion strategy into real-world, clinical benefits. Evaluation of combined reperfusion strategies must consider the individual risks of each component of pharmacoinvasive therapy in selecting appropriate target populations, study protocols, and endpoints. This chapter will provide an overview of central issues in modern-day clinical trials of pharmacoinvasive therapy for ST segment elevation myocardial infarction (STEMI) as well as a review of previous, ongoing, and terminated trials, with an emphasis on trial design and the challenges facing clinical design in this arena.

II. TRIALS OF PHARMACOINVASIVE THERAPY

As discussed in previous chapters, the principle of pharmacoinvasive therapy is to combine medical and mechanical therapies in order to optimize the likelihood of successful reperfusion in STEMI. Fundamentally, the marriage of three concepts drives clinical trial efforts of pharmacoinvasive therapy. First, "time is myocardium," regardless of whether the therapeutic strategy is fibrinolysis (2) or mechanical reperfusion (3). Second, primary percutaneous coronary intervention (PCI) appears to be superior to fibrinolysis (4) and, as such, should be extended to as many patients with STEMI as is feasible. Third, among patients undergoing primary PCI, spontaneous reperfusion prior to definitive mechanical revascularization powerfully predicts improved outcomes. Data from 2507 pooled patients in the four Primary Angioplasty in Myocardial Infarction (PAMI) trials demonstrates that pre-procedural normal Thrombolysis in Myocardial Infarction (TIMI) grade 3 flow in the infarct-related artery (IRA) is an independent predictor of early and late survival, even when corrected for postprocedural flow grade (5).

The goal of clinical trials of pharmacoinvasive therapy is to determine the ideal combination of upstream medical adjuvant therapy for percutaneous coronary intervention. Candidate regimens have included full-dose fibrinolytic + percutaneous coronary intervention (PCI), reduced-dose fibrinolytic + glycoprotein receptor (GP) IIb/IIIa antagonists ("Combination Therapy") + PCI, and GP IIb/IIIa alone with PCI (Table 8.1). Additional areas of investigation include the dosing and use of antithrombins such as unfractionated heparin (UFH), low molecular weight heparins (LMWH), and direct thrombin inhibitors (DTI), as well as synergistic antiplatelet therapy with thienopyridines.

A. Early Trials Combining Balloon Angioplasty and Fibrinolysis

The theoretically complementary features of medical and invasive reperfusion strategies led to pilot studies of combined medical and mechanical reperfusion therapy, but early results were disappointing. O'Neill et al. found a higher rate of severe bleeding complications, longer and more expensive hospital stays, and an increased need for

Table 8.1 Contemporary Trials of Pharmacoinvasive Therapy

Trial	n	GP IIb/IIIa	Fibrinolytic	Arms of therapy	Anti-thrombin	Primary endpoint	Status
ADVANCE-MI	148 (5640)	Eptifibatide	Tenecteplase	GP IIb/IIIa + PCI; GP IIb/IIIa + RDL + PCI	UFH vs. enoxaparin	Death + MI + severe CHF at 30 days	Terminated
ASSENT 4	4000	Not specified	Tenecteplase	FDL + PCI; PCI	UFH	Death + cardiogenic shock + CHF at 90 days	Ongoing
BRAVE	253	Abciximab	Reteplase	GP IIb/IIIa + PCI; GP IIb/IIIa + RDL + PCI	UFH	Infarct size by SPECT at 5–10 days	Completed
CAPITAL MI	170	None	Tenecteplase	FDL; FDL + PCI	UFH	Death + MI + stroke + recurrent ischemia at 30 days	Completed
FINESSE	3000	Abciximab	Reteplase	GP IIb/IIIa (ED) + PCI; GP Ib/IIIa (Lab) + PCI; GP IIb/IIIa + RDL + PCI	UFH vs. enoxaparin	Death + VF + CHF + cardiogenic shock at 90 days	Ongoing

ED, emergency department; FDL, full-dose fibrinolytic; GP IIb/IIIa, glycoprotein receptor IIb/IIIa antagonist; Lab, cardiac catheterization laboratory; MI, myocardial infarction; PCI, percutaneous coronary intervention; RDL, reduced-dose fibrinolytic; UFH, unfractionated heparin.

emergent coronary artery bypass graft (CABG) surgery in a randomized trial of 122 patients receiving intravenous streptokinase with planned primary angioplasty or angioplasty alone for STEMI (6). The Thrombolysis and Angioplasty in Acute Myocardial Infarction (TAMI) Study Group treated 386 STEMI patients with intravenous (IV) alteplase (t-PA) and performed routine angiography at 90 minutes. Those with TIMI grade 2–3 epicardial flow but >50% residual stenoses were randomized to immediate or delayed angioplasty. In this trial, patients who underwent early angioplasty suffered excess mortality and had higher rates of CABG surgery, urgent repeat angioplasty, and severe bleeding (7). Similarly, in an investigation performed by the European Cooperative Study Group, 367 patients with STEMI who received IV t-PA were randomized to angioplasty or noninvasive strategies for STEMI. Early intervention was associated with higher mortality as well as more bleeding, hypotension, and recurrent ischemia (8). The TIMI Study Group randomized 586 patients with STEMI to treatment with t-PA plus immediate catheterization and angioplasty, delayed catheterization and angioplasty, or medical therapy in the TIMI IIa trial. Of the three arms, those who underwent immediate intervention suffered the highest rate of the combined study endpoint of death or myocardial infarction (MI) at 6 weeks (9). Together, these early trials suggested that full-dose fibrinolysis was incompatible with balloon angioplasty.

B.   Initial Studies of Pharmacoinvasive Therapy

New developments in medical therapies paved the way for pharmacoinvasive therapy. Efforts to improve pharmacological reperfusion strategies resulted in discoveries about the central role of platelets (10), platelet glycoprotein (GP) IIb/IIIa antagonists (11), and optimal (lower) UFH dosing. Simultaneous improvements in interventional techniques, catheters, stents, and other devices expanded upon balloon angioplasty to produce the modern lesion-specific PCI approach in interventional cardiology (12). These parallel advances led investigators to reconsider the incompatibility of full-dose fibrinolysis and primary PCI.

   In the Plasminogen-activator Angioplasty Compatibility Trial (PACT), 606 patients with STEMI were randomized to placebo or reduced-dose recombinant tissue plasminogen activator (rt-PA) in the context of universal aspirin, UFH, and immediate catheterization. Although patent arteries (TIMI grade 2 or 3 flow) on diagnostic catheterization were significantly more frequent with recombinant t-PA therapy than placebo, treatment assignment did not impact initial or convalescent ventricular function (13). Importantly, angioplasty procedural success was not diminished by pretreatment with rt-PA (92.8% rt-PA vs. 94.6% placebo; $p = 0.52$), and adverse events including stroke (0.7% rt-PA vs. 0.7% placebo; $p = 0.99$), major hemorrhage (8.5% vs. 8.2%; $p = 0.092$), intracranial hemorrhage (0.3% vs. 0.3%; $p = 0.99$), in-hospital mortality (3.6% vs. 3.0%; $p = 0.62$), and 30-day mortality (3.6% vs. 3.3%; $p = 0.81$) were not more frequent. Thus, reduced-dose fibrinolytic therapy before primary PCI appeared to be reasonably safe and associated with improved IRA flow.

Similarly, in the Strategies for Patency Enhancement in the Emergency Department (SPEED) trial, patients with STEMI were randomized to receive full-dose reteplase, abciximab, or combination therapy with reduced-dose reteplase + abciximab followed by immediate diagnostic catheterization. The primary endpoint, the rate of TIMI grade 3 flow at 60–90 minutes, was improved with the combination reteplase (5 U + 5 U) + abciximab + standard dose UFH when compared with standard dose reteplase (10 U + 10 U) + standard dose UFH (61.1% vs. 46.9%; $p = 0.05$) (14). Although the subsequent performance of PCI was neither randomized nor mandated, patients who were treated with combination therapy had improved pre-PCI infarct artery flow, improved procedural success, and trends toward decreases in death, reinfarction, and urgent revascularization compared with those patients who received full-dose reteplase or abciximab alone before primary PCI.

C. Contemporary Trials of Pharmacoinvasive Therapy

One randomized trial in which patients with STEMI received therapy with GP IIb/IIIa blockade alone or GP IIb/IIIa blockade + reduced-dose fibrinolysis with a planned early invasive strategy has been reported: the Bavarian Revascularization Alternatives (BRAVE) Trial. The principal hypothesis in this trial was that upstream combination therapy with reduced-dose fibrinolytics + GP IIb/IIIa blockade + primary PCI would result in smaller scintigraphic infarct size when compared with upstream GP IIb/IIIa blockade + primary PCI. Two hundred fifty-three patients with acute STEMI were randomized to therapy with abciximab + PCI or abciximab + reduced-dose reteplase + PCI. While pre-PCI TIMI grade 3 flow was higher among patients treated with combination therapy (TIMI III flow 40% vs. 18%; $p < 0.01$), scintigraphic infarct size was not reduced in the combination therapy arm versus the abciximab alone (13% vs. 11.5%, respectively; $p = 0.81$) (15). There were nonsignificant increases in death/MI (2.4% vs. 1.6%), death/MI/stroke (3.2% vs. 1.6%), and major bleeding (5.6% vs. 1.6%) with combination therapy. Subset analyses of patients who required transfer for primary PCI and those who had earlier times to revascularization revealed no differences.

The findings from the BRAVE trial should be interpreted cautiously, as this was a small trial that was significantly underpowered to show differences in clinical endpoints and infarct size with SPECT sestabimi scanning has not been proven to be a reliable surrogate biomarker to differentiate the benefits of therapies for STEMI. As discussed in previous chapters, combination therapy with GP IIb/IIIa receptor blockade and fibrinolysis has been shown to improve surrogate biomarkers such as angiographic flow patterns and ST segment resolution in randomized clinical trials (14, 16–18). However, combination medical therapy without immediate PCI was not shown to improve survival in two large studies (19,20). Thus, the relationship between surrogate biomarkers of reperfusion success and clinical outcomes such as mortality is uncertain, so the risks and benefits of pharmacoinvasive are best studied in large-scale, definitive trials that are adequately powered to detect differences in clinical outcomes. The Facilitated INtervention with Enhanced Reperfusion Speed to Stop Events (FINESSE) trial is the single ongoing trial studying combination pharmacoinvasive therapy for STEMI (21). Three arms of therapy will be compared in a 1:1:1 fashion in 3000 patients:

- Early PCI after reduced-dose reteplase (5 U +5 U) + abciximab bolus doses administered in the emergency department
- Early PCI after abciximab bolus administered in the emergency department
- Primary PCI with abciximab initiated in the cardiac catheterization lab (Fig. 8.1)

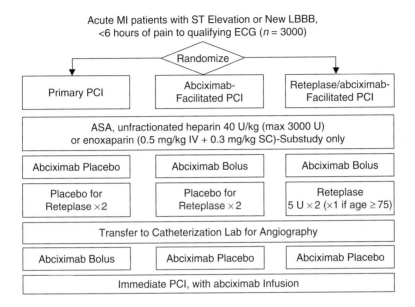

Figure 8.1 FINESSE trial design. (From Herrmann HC, Kelley MP, Ellis SG. J Invasive Cardiol. 2001.)

The primary efficacy endpoint of FINESSE is the composite of all-cause mortality and post-MI complications within 90 days of randomization. Complications included in the endpoint are resuscitated ventricular fibrillation occurring >48 hours after randomization, rehospitalization or emergency department visit for congestive heart failure, and cardiogenic shock. This composite endpoint was chosen to reflect the physiological hypothesis that combination medical therapy prior to PCI will result in earlier and improved reperfusion, leading to improved myocardial salvage and, hence, decreased infarct size-dependent complications.

The estimates used to create the composite endpoint were based on previous clinical trials of STEMI [death (4–6%), cardiogenic shock (5–7%), late resuscitated VF (0.5–2%) and rehospitalization for HF (4–7%)], acknowledging some overlap for infarct size-related complications. Risk groups were divided into low, medium, and high based on time-to-treatment data from clinical trials and registry data to assist in power calculations. Using these estimates, FINESSE will have ≥80% power to detect a difference in the primary endpoint between the pharmacoinvasive strategy and the primary PCI strategy at a statistical significance level of $p \leq 0.05$ using a two-sided log-rank test. The relative risk reduction in low-risk patients is estimated to be 15%, in medium-risk patients 25%, and in high-risk patients 35%. Extensive prespecified subgroup analyses will be performed based on traditional and novel risk factors for adverse outcomes. FINESSE will include a site-level randomized substudy wherein prespecified sites will use enoxaparin in place of low-dose UFH to evaluate its utility in pharmacoinvasive therapy. It is anticipated that approximately 1000 of the 3000 enrolled will participate in the enoxaparin substudy.

While FINESSE and BRAVE have focused upon combination therapy in conjunction with early PCI, other trials are focusing instead upon full-dose thrombolytic therapy as part of the pharmacoinvasive approach (Table 8.1). In the recently presented Combined Angioplasty and Pharmacological Intervention versus Thrombolysis Alone in Acute Myocardial Infarction (CAPITAL-AMI) trial, 170 high-risk MI patients from four referral centers in Ottawa were randomized to fibrinolysis alone with full-dose tenecteplase (TNK) or fibrinolysis with full-dose TNK followed by immediate transfer to a single referral center for acute angiography and possible PCI (pharmacoinvasive group). In the fibrinolysis-alone group, if reperfusion was successful, patients were given standard follow-up care, but if reperfusion was unsuccessful, patients were transferred for angiography and possible intervention to the same referral center. The primary endpoint was the composite of death, MI, stroke, or recurrent ischemia at 30 days, which was significantly reduced in the combination group (9.3% in pharmacoinvasive group vs. 21.4% in fibrinolysis alone group; $p = 0.034$) (22). The incidence of TIMI major bleeding was similar (9.3% vs. 8.3%, respectively; $p =$ NS). Trends were seen toward reduced length of stay, decreased cardiogenic shock, and decreased heart failure among the pharmacoinvasive group. This small study suggests the feasibility of combining TNK with primary PCI and will likely spark enrollment in the ongoing ASSENT-4 study.

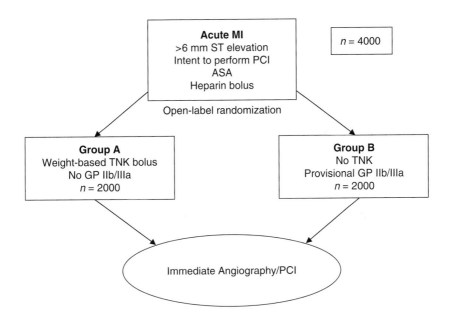

Figure 8.2   ASSENT-4 trial design.

The Assessment of the Safety and Efficacy of a New Thrombolytic Regimen (ASSENT)–4 trial is an ongoing trial combining fibrinolysis with primary PCI, although GP IIb/IIIa blockade use is not mandated in this protocol. Four thousand patients with STEMI will be treated with aspirin and UFH and randomized to upstream TNK therapy prior to PCI (Group A) versus routine primary PCI (Group B) (C. Granger, Personal Communication, 2004). The use of GP IIb/IIIa is prohibited among patients assigned to Group A, whereas provisional use is allowed at the discretion of the investigator in Group B (Fig. 8.2). The primary endpoint in this trial is the 90-day composite of death, cardiogenic shock, or congestive heart failure.

This trial aims to include a high-risk population by requiring a total of at least 6 mm of ST segment elevation on the qualifying electrocardiogram and by excluding patients who are anticipated to arrive at the catheterization laboratory within 60 minutes of randomization. There is no upper age limit. However, there are no dose alterations for the elderly in this trial, though heparin dosing is lower among patients who will receive TNK. Target-activated clotting times are also lower among patients who receive provisional GP IIb/IIIa blockade.

The ADdressing the Value of Facilitated ANgioplasty Compared with Eptifibatide Monotherapy in Acute Myocardial Infarction (ADVANCE MI) trial, another large pharmacoinvasive trial, began enrolling patients in October 2002. This study was designed to randomize 5640 patients with STEMI to eptifibatide monotherapy or eptifibatide with reduced-dose TNK combination therapy prior to primary PCI. A subrandomization of enoxaparin or unfractionated heparin was planned in a 2×2 fashion. However, after enrollment of fewer than 3% of intended subjects over 11 months, the trial was discontinued not for reasons related to safety or efficacy, but rather because the trial was felt not to be executable in its intended form. Some investigators noted that they perceived divergent pressures: brisk enrollment vs. institutional efforts to shorten "door-to-balloon" times that may have been limited by the time delays associated with obtaining informed consent, randomization, and other vital protocol measures. Similar to the AIR-PAMI experience, patient accrual was slower than anticipated, resulting in premature termination. The ethical implications of premature termination of a trial for reasons other than achievement of a prespecified endpoint are considerable and have been discussed elsewhere (23). However, given increasing financial pressures on hospitals and the increased scrutiny through quality monitoring by reimbursement and accreditation agencies, clinical trials of pharmacoinvasive therapy will need to be adapted to contemporary clinical practice with efficient consent and randomization processes.

III. KEY ISSUES IN PHARMACOINVASIVE THERAPY TRIALS

The rationale for pharmacoinvasive therapy has been extensively discussed in the preceding chapters. While primary PCI appears superior to fibrinolytic therapy for STEMI when performed in a timely fashion by experienced operators in high-volume centers, the optimal medical adjunctive therapies for primary PCI have not been clearly defined. Furthermore, emerging data suggest that transfer strategies for primary PCI may be preferable to on-site fibrinolysis strategies (4). Unfortunately, only a minority of the U.S. population is served by hospital centers with invasive capabilities. Among the 1506 hospitals participating in the National Registry of Myocardial Infarction (NRMI)-2, 39.2% of hospitals in the United States have PCI capability with surgical backup, while an additional 7.4% are PCI-capable but lack surgical backup (24). Previous, more conservative estimates placed the number of PCI-capable centers at 20% nationwide, with centers concentrated in urban and suburban locations (25). This geographic discrepancy underscores the need to study combination medical therapies that could extend the window of opportunity for patients to receive mechanical reperfusion beyond the currently recommended 90-minute time frame, by allowing patients to be safely transported to invasive centers after initial stabilization.

Important considerations in trials of pharmacoinvasive strategies for STEMI include (a) careful selection of the appropriate target population, including the elderly and patients who require transfer to an invasive center, (b) determination of an acceptable time delay to invasive therapy, especially considering the policy complexity of interhospital transfer, (c) proactive steps to reduce risks of hemorrhagic complications, and (d) measurement of the appropriate endpoints.

A. What Is the Target Population?

Patients with the greatest potential to derive benefits from pharmacoinvasive reperfusion are those who are at the highest risk of poor outcomes. Predictors of poor outcomes in STEMI include advanced age, presentation with signs of heart failure or cardiogenic shock, significant time delay to presentation or atypical symptoms causing delayed diagnosis of STEMI, female gender, low body weight, renal insufficiency, and significant comorbidity, among other factors (26,27). Paradoxically, trial subject selection criteria have tended to exclude many such patients, in particular the elderly, for unclear reasons

(28,29), despite evidence that the elderly are not less likely to be willing to participate (30). Further, even when high-risk patients are not frankly excluded, hesitation by site investigators to enroll such patients may cause ascertainment bias, which ultimately limits the applicability of trial findings to the real-world setting. However, to exclude such high-risk patients in a study is to potentially blunt a therapeutic advantage that a more aggressive strategy may provide.

From a trial-design and statistical perspective, the inclusion of higher-risk patients creates a higher event rate in the control arm. This may allow for a smaller sample size to achieve the same power to detect a given therapeutic effect, and therefore may be more cost-effective than studying a larger sample of lower-risk subjects. The issues surrounding the selection of target patients are complex and require careful consideration. The FINESSE protocol actively seeks a high-risk population by excluding patients who are less than 60 years of age with localized inferior infarction as well as those who have anticipated times to arrival in the catheterization laboratory of fewer than 60 minutes. Both FINESSE and ADVANCE MI specifically did not exclude patients with cardiogenic shock or advanced age.

B. Is Pharmacoinvasive Therapy Only for Transfer Patients?

Patients who initially present to centers without invasive capabilities potentially constitute a group particularly well suited to benefit from pharmacoinvasive strategies. It is clear that prolonged door-to-balloon times are associated with poor outcomes (31), and among more than 40,000 patients studied in the NRMI-3, the most potent predictor of prolonged door-to-balloon times was interhospital transfer (32). However, transfer strategies require integrated logistical planning, which may be complicated. Referring centers need clearly defined protocols for upstream medical stabilization as well as smooth communication systems to ensure that receiving centers are continuously aware of the status of a given patient and are able to rapidly activate the catheterization laboratory in anticipation of patient arrival.

Dedication to overcome such hurdles can extend preferable, previously unavailable therapy further into the community. The notion of a hub-and-spoke model wherein referring centers without invasive capabilities—spokes—rapidly assess, stabilize, and transfer patients with STEMI to regional invasive centers—hubs—has been gaining momentum as the advantages of primary PCI over on-site fibrinolysis have become better understood (33,34). While there are limited clinical trial data from the United States (AIR PAMI), data from European trials such as the Danish Multicenter Randomized Study on Fibrinolytic Therapy versus Acute Coronary ANgioplasty in Acute Myocardial Infarction (DANAMI-2) trial (35), the PRimary Angioplasty in AMI Patients From General Community Hospitals Transported to PTCA Units vs. Emergency Thrombolysis (PRAGUE) trial (36), and the PRAGUE-2 trial (37), as well as meta-analysis (4), suggest that transfer for primary PCI may be superior to on-site fibrinolysis in reducing rates of fatal MI, stroke, and death/MI/stroke despite inherent prolongations in time to reperfusion. However, even at invasive centers, other factors such as time of day, weekend-versus-weekday presentation, and PCI volume of the receiving center powerfully predict prolonged door-to-balloon times (32). FINESSE explicitly targets patients who are to be transferred for primary PCI with a goal enrollment of 50% of interhospital transfer patients.

C. What Is an Acceptable Delay for Primary PCI or Pharmacoinvasive Therapy?

Present ACC/AHA guidelines for the management of acute myocardial infarction recommend delays of not longer than 90 (±30) minutes from admission to balloon inflation for primary PCI (38). However, the clinical reality is that average door-to-balloon in the recent NRMI-3 registry was just over 2 hours at primary PCI centers and over 3 hours for patients transferred from a community hospital to a tertiary hospital for primary PCI (32). Therefore, administration of potent adjunctive pharmacological agents at the time of initial presentation may be synergistic and help overcome the delays inherent in reperfusion when transferring patients for primary PCI. Furthermore, up to 20% of patients taken to the lab with the intent of primary PCI do not receive it secondary to anatomical limitations. This population may also derive clinical benefit from a more potent medical regimen.

Table 8.2 Median Time Intervals for Patients Randomly Assigned to Transfer for Primary Percutaneous Coronary Intervention

Study (Ref.)	Time Interval (min) Door to randomization	Randomization to departure	Transfer time	Door to balloon[a]	Symptom onset to balloon
PRAGUE-1 (10) (n = 101)	15	17	35	28	215
PRAGUE-2 (11) (n = 429)	20	NR	48	26	277
DANAMI-2 (9) (n = 567)	22	38	32	26	224
AIR-PAMI (12) (n = 71)	35	38	26	25	NR

NR = not reported.
[a] Time from arrival at tertiary hospital until first balloon inflation during PCI.
Source: Ref. 34.

The guidelines predate data from trials in which times longer than 90 minutes have outperformed primary fibrinolysis. In DANAMI-2, up to 3 hours was allowed for transfer according to the protocol, though the median time for transport was substantially shorter at 63 minutes; transfer accounted for ~14% of total time from symptom onset to reperfusion. The median total time from randomization to first balloon inflation was 90 minutes, with a median of 22 minutes from presentation to randomization (35) (Table 8.2).

In the only comparable U.S. trial of such a strategy, the Air Primary Angioplasty in Myocardial Infarction (AIR PAMI) study, door-to-balloon times were 155 minutes, including 35 minutes from presentation to randomization. Unfortunately, this promising study was terminated early secondary to slow patient accrual. Point estimates favoring transfer for primary PCI over on-site fibrinolysis were seen among the 138 patients who were randomized, with major adverse cardiac events (death, reinfarction, or stroke) occurring in 8.4% of patients treated with PCI versus 13.6% of patients treated with fibrinolysis

(p = 0.331) (39), although these findings were not statistically significant. In both the AIR-PAMI and DANAMI-2 trials, patients randomized to primary PCI were treated with aspirin and UFH, a regimen associated with very poor spontaneous reperfusion rates (40).

By adding a glycoprotein IIb/IIIa antagonist ± fibrinolytic, modern pharmacoinvasive trials may be able to justify studying a longer window of opportunity by increasing the rate of spontaneous reperfusion before undergoing definitive revascularization. Both FINESSE and ADVANCE MI empirically chose 4 hours as the acceptable upper time limit for inclusion, whereas ASSENT-4 chose 3 hours. Both FINESSE and ASSENT-4 also have lower time limits of 1 hour; patients with very short times to PCI have "early reperfusion" by definition and would likely derive no additional benefit but would likely experience increased bleeding risks. Ultimately, time to reperfusion cannot be reliably predicted before primary PCI, so the "acceptable delay" for pharmacoinvasive therapy will be defined retrospectively from data collected in trials and registries of STEMI as that which results in overall outcomes not worse than on-site fibrinolysis.

D. Can Bleeding Risk Be Minimized in Pharmacoinvasive Reperfusion?

Findings from the Global Utilization of Strategies to Open Occluded Arteries (GUSTO) V and Assessment of the Safety and Efficacy of a New Thrombolytic Regimen (ASSENT)-3 trials suggest that with more aggressive antithrombotic therapy, there are increased risks of bleeding. In both trials, transfusions, thrombocytopenia, and mild, moderate, and severe bleeding — including intracranial hemorrhage (ICH) and spontaneous nonintracranial hemorrhage — were all more common among patients treated with combination reduced-dose fibrinolytic and GP IIb/IIIa blockade than among those treated with full-dose fibrinolytic and UFH, despite lower median partial thromboplastin times. Of particular concern, elderly patients were found to have three times the rate of ICH with combination therapy than fibrinolytic alone in ASSENT-3 (13.3% vs. 4.1%) (20). In GUSTO V, patients >75 years old had a trend toward an increased risk of ICH with combination therapy (2.1% vs. 1.1%; p = 0.069), and there was a significant interaction for treatment by age <75 or ≥75 years for intracranial hemorrhage (p = 0.033) (19).

In order to minimize the increased risk of bleeding complications, modern pharmacoinvasive trials have down-adjusted heparin nomograms and prescribed lower doses of study drugs for elder patients. For example, in FINESSE, patients aged >75 years will receive a novel single half-dose (5 U) of reteplase in combination with abciximab, and all patients will receive very low-dose heparin (40 U/kg bolus). Similarly, one of the key features planned in the ADVANCE MI study was testing the hypothesis that reduced-dose antithrombotics in the elderly might lower the risk of combination therapy while preserving or even increasing efficacy. Consequently, the ADVANCE MI protocol had dose adjustments to all study drugs for patients ≥75 years of age.

E. What Endpoints Should Be Used in Pharmacoinvasive Trials?

The selection of suitable endpoints for pharmacoinvasive therapy trials is a complex issue. The caveats of surrogate endpoints have been illustrated by the failure of promising combination medical therapies to produce mortality reductions in phase III trials after favorable findings in phase II trials. For example, the SPEED study suggested that combination therapy with reteplase plus abciximab improved the incidence of early (between 60 and 90 min) TIMI grade 3 flow rates when compared to reteplase alone in acute STEMI. However, when the same agents were compared in GUSTO V, a mortality study, combination therapy was not found to be superior to fibrinolytic alone, and while noninferior, combination therapy came at a cost of an increased rate of non-intracranial hemorrhage. Given the increased risks of major and minor bleeding, there is an onus to demonstrate that advanced combination therapies impart meaningful clinical benefits to offset the risk. Consequently, the role of surrogate endpoints is limited in this context. As such, trials of pharmacoinvasive therapy should be designed around the power to detect differences in clinical outcomes of STEMI, such as death, stroke, heart failure, and cardiogenic shock. Thus, "net clinical benefit" strategies for endpoints, such as those that combine both safety and efficacy endpoints, are a reasonable approach as they are patient-focused in defining useful therapy. One such example of a net clinical benefit was employed in the recent Randomized Evaluation in PCI

Linking Angiomax to Reduced Clinical Events (REPLACE)-2 trial in elective or urgent PCI, in which bivalirudin plus provisional GP IIb/IIIa was found not to be inferior to UFH and routine GP IIb/IIIa therapy with a quadruple primary endpoint of 30-day death, MI, or urgent repeat revascularization, or in-hospital major bleeding (41).

F.   Is There a Role for Prehospital Fibrinolysis?

In an effort to improve symptom onset-to-reperfusion times, several clinical trials have investigated the utility of hospital evaluation and therapy to speed STEMI care. The feasibility of prehospital electrocardiogram acquisition has been well demonstrated and is estimated to add minimal time to the time required for transportation (42,43). Observations from NRMI-2 suggest that the time to treatment is lowered with prehospital electrocardiography (10-min decrease in door-to-medication time, 23-min decrease in door-to-balloon times) (44). With ever-improving mobile and wireless technology, the barriers to acquisition and transmission of EKGs to destination care centers are rapidly diminishing. Present ACC/AHA guidelines for acute myocardial infarction support prehospital evaluation and diagnosis, including electrocardiography.

Meta-analysis of six trials of prehospital fibrinolysis including 6434 patients suggests that its use is associated with a substantial reduction in time to treat (58 min) and a 17% relative risk reduction of mortality (45). However, these studies were largely performed in European centers with mobile care units staffed by physicians and nurses experienced in the administration of fibrinolytic therapy, a scenario uncommon in American care systems. Therefore, the applicability of such findings is limited in the United States.

The recently described international ASSENT-3 plus trial evaluated the safety and efficacy of prehospital fibrinolysis with TNK + enoxaparin and TNK + UFH versus historical controls from ASSENT-3. In the former study, the primary efficacy endpoint of the 30-day incidence of death, myocardial infarction, or in-hospital refractory ischemia tended to favor the enoxaparin group, although the results did not achieve statistical significance (14.2% vs. 17.4%; $p = 0.08$) (46). The efficacy and safety endpoint was the composite of the efficacy endpoint with in-hospital major bleeding or intracranial hemorrhage and was similar across treatment groups (18.3% for enoxaparin vs. 20.3% for UFH; $p = 0.297$). In-hospital recurrent MI was less common among patients treated with enoxaparin (3.55% vs. 5.85%; $p = 0.028$), and there was a nonsignificant trend favoring refractory ischemia. Collapsing across treatment groups, median time to treatment was 45 minutes shorter from symptom onset to TNK injection in ASSENT-3 plus than in ASSENT-3. However, these salutary effects were counterbalanced by an excess of stroke (2.93% with enoxaparin vs. 1.34% with UFH; $p = 0.026$) and an excess of ICH (2.2% vs. 0.97%; $p = 0.047$). Among patients >75 years of age, ICH occurred in nearly 7% assigned to enoxaparin vs. fewer than 1% of patients assigned UFH.

Prehospital TNK + UFH was found to be as safe and efficacious as when administered in the hospital, and prehospital treatment in high-risk patients resulted in the same mortality rates as in-hospital treatment in low-risk patients, suggesting that it may be a promising strategy. These findings have important implications for pharmacoinvasive protocols, with specific regard to safety. Whereas TNK + enoxaparin was found to be superior to TNK + UFH when administered in-hospital with regard to both safety and efficacy, the opposite safety profile was found in prehospital therapy. This suggests that acute transport may make dosing of medications more challenging and safety more difficult to predict. Careful attention must be paid to assumptions that superior in-hospital regimens will remain superior when administered outside the hospital setting. Because of complex medical, legal, and social interactions, prehospital fibrinolysis has not been recommended outside specific circumstances, such as prolonged transport times and physician presence. Given the rarity of such systems in the United States, clinical trials of pharmacoinvasive therapy reliant upon resource-heavy prehospital care would not be readily applicable in the United States and therefore are not a large part of the landscape.

IV. THE POTENTIAL IMPACT OF A POSITIVE PHARMACOINVASIVE REPERFUSION TRIAL

Pharmacoinvasive therapy is likely to prove to be beneficial for certain groups of patients with STEMI. Patients with high-risk presentations who are likely to have prolonged times to mechanical reperfusion or those whose care is limited by logistic or geographic considerations stand the greatest chance to derive a benefit. If trials of pharmacoinvasive therapy are successful in defining subgroups that derive substantial benefits, there would be added grounds for the creation of regional care networks akin to trauma care, whereby patients are rapidly stabilized and triaged to locally defined centers of excellence for the invasive portion of pharmacoinvasive therapy for STEMI. Support for this type of approach in the literature is increasing, with several recent editorials calling for standardization of triage systems and nomenclature (33,34,47).

V. SUMMARY AND CONCLUSIONS

Pharmacoinvasive therapy is a compelling concept, but as yet there are limited definite data to support its utility. Whereas early trials evaluating combination therapy were disappointing, subsequent studies have suggested that not only are combination therapy and mechanical revascularization compatible, but their coupling may be preferable for certain groups. However, unlike the near-universal benefits of aspirin, the utility of pharmacoinvasive therapy may be limited to an as-yet-unidentified niche of high-risk STEMI patients. The successful application of this idea will require an understanding of the lessons from previous trials of similar therapy and intelligent formulation of subsequent questions. Unfortunately, because of the complex current environment of STEMI care, there are only two large ongoing trials of pharmacoinvasive therapy. The premature termination of the ADVANCE-MI and related AIR-PAMI trials underscores the challenges in executing a pharmacoinvasive trial of STEMI, but the potential impact of a positive trial remains vast.

REFERENCES

1. Dauerman HL, Sobel, BE. Synergistic treatment of ST segment elevation myocardial infarction with pharmacoinvasive recanalization. J Am Coll Cardiol 2003; 42: 646–651.

2. Newby LK, Rutsch WR, Califf RM, et al. Time from symptom onset to treatment and outcomes after thrombolytic therapy. J Am Coll Cardiol 1996;27:1646–1655.

3. De Luca G, Suryapranata H, Ottervanger JP, Antman EM. Time delay to treatment and mortality in primary angioplasty for acute myocardial infarction: every minute of delay counts. Circulation 2004;109(10): 1223–1225.

4. Keeley EC, Boura JA, Grines CL. Primary angioplasty versus intravenous thrombolytic therapy for acute myocardial infarction: a quantitative review of 23 randomised trials. Lancet 2003;361:13–20

5. Stone GW, Cox D, Garcia E, Brodie BR, Morice MC, Griffin J, Mattos L, Lansky AJ, O'Neill WW, Grines CL. Normal flow (TIMI 3) before mechanical reperfusion therapy is an independent determinant of survival in acute myocardial infarction: analysis from the primary angioplasty in myocardial infarction trials. Circulation 2001;104(6): 636–641.

6. O'Neill WW, Weintraub R, Grines CL, Meany TB, Brodie BR, Friedman HZ, Ramos RG, Gangadharan V, Levin RN, Choksi N, et al. A prospective, placebo-controlled, randomized trial of intravenous streptokinase and angioplasty versus lone angioplasty therapy of acute myocardial infarction. Circulation 1992;86(6):1710–1717.

7. Topol EJ, Califf RM, George BS, et al., and the Thrombolysis and Angioplasty in Acute Myocardial Infarction Study Group. A randomized trial of immediate vs. delayed elective angioplasty after intravenous tissue plasminogen activator in acute myocardial infarction. N Engl J Med 1987;317:581–588.

8. Simoons ML, Arnold AE, Betriu A, et al., for the European Cooperative Study Group for recombinant tissue-type plasminogen activator (rTPA). Thrombolysis with tissue plasminogen activator in acute myocardial infarction: no additional benefit from immediate percutaneous coronary angioplasty. Lancet 1988;1:197–203.

9. The TIMI Research Group. Immediate versus delayed catheterization and angioplasty following thrombolytic therapy for acute myocardial infarction. TIMI IIa results. JAMA 1988;206:2849–2858.

10. Topol EJ. Toward a new frontier in myocardial reperfusion therapy: emerging platelet preeminence. Circulation 1998;97(2):211–218.

11. Brener SJ et al. on behalf of the Reopro and primary PTCA organization and randomized trial (RAPPORT) investigators. Randomized, placebo-controlled trial of primary glycoprotein IIb/IIIa blockade with primary angioplasty for acute MI. Circulation 1998;98:734–741.

12. Smith SC, Jr, Dove JT, Jacobs AK, Kennedy JW, Kereiakes D, Kern MJ, Kuntz RE, Popma JJ, Schaff HV, Williams DO. ACC/AHA guidelines for percutaneous coronary intervention: a report of the American College of Cardiology/American Heart Association Task Force on Practice Guidelines (Committee to Revise the 1993 Guidelines for Percutaneous Transluminal Coronary Angioplasty). J Am Coll Cardiol 2001; 37:2239.

13. Ross AM, Coyne KS, Reiner JS, et al. A randomized trial comparing primary angioplasty with a strategy of short-acting thrombolysis and immediate planned rescue angioplasty in acute myocardial infarction: The PACT trial. J Am Coll Cardiol 1999;34:1954–1962.

14. SPEED Group. Trial of abciximab with and without low-dose reteplase for acute myocardial infarction. Circulation 2000;101:2788–2794.

15. Kastrati A, Mehilli J, Schlotterbeck K, Dotzer F, Dirschinger J, Schmitt C, Nekolla SG, Seyfarth M, Martinoff S, Markwardt C, Clermont G, Gerbig HW, Leiss J, Schwaiger M, Schomig A; Bavarian Reperfusion Alternatives Evaluation (BRAVE) Study Investigators. Early administration of reteplase plus abciximab vs. abciximab alone in patients with acute myocardial infarction referred for percutaneous coronary intervention: a randomized controlled trial. JAMA 2004;291(8):947–954.

16. Antman EM, Giugliano RP, Gibson CM, et al., for the TIMI Investigators. Abciximab facilitates the rate and extent of thrombolysis: Results of the Thrombolysis in Myocardial Infarction (TIMI) 14 Trial. Circulation 1999;99:2720–2732.

17. Brener SJ, Zeymer U, Adgey J, et al., for the INTRO AMI Investigators. Eptifibatide and low-dose tissue plasminogen activator in acute myocardial infarction: the Integrilin and Low Dose Thrombolysis in Acute Myocardial Infarction (INTRO AMI) Trial. J Am Coll Cardiol 2002;39: 377–386.

18. Giugliano RP, Roe MT, Harrington RA, Gibson CM, Zeymer U, Van de Werf F, Baran KW, Hobbach HP, Woodlief LH, Hannan KL, Greenberg S, Miller J, Kitt MM, Strony J, McCabe CH, Braunwald E, Califf

RM; INTEGRITI Investigators. Combination reperfusion therapy with eptifibatide and reduced-dose tenecteplase for ST-elevation myocardial infarction: results of the integrilin and tenecteplase in acute myocardial infarction (INTEGRITI) Phase II Angiographic Trial. J Am Coll Cardiol 2003;41(8):1251–1260.

19. The GUSTO Investigators. Reperfusion therapy for acute myocardial infarction with fibrinolytic therapy or combination reduced fibrinolytic therapy and platelet glycoprotein IIb/IIIa inhibition: the GUSTO V randomised trial. Lancet 2001;357:1905–1914.

20. The ASSENT-3 Investigators. Efficacy and safety of tenecteplase in combination with enoxaparin, abciximab, or unfractionated heparin: the ASSENT-3 randomised trial in acute myocardial infarction. Lancet 2001;358:605–613.

21. Herrmann HC, Kelley MP, Ellis SG. Facilitated PCI: rationale and design of the FINESSE trial. J Invasive Cardiol 2001;13 (suppl A): 10A–15A.

22. Le May M, Michel LeMay, for the CAPITAL AMI Investigators. Combined Angioplasty and Pharmacological Intervention versus Thrombolysis Alone in Acute Myocardial Infarction (CAPITAL-AMI) trial. Presented at ACC Scientific Sessions, New Orleans, LA, March 8, 2004.

23. Psaty BM, Rennie D. Stopping medical research to save money: a broken pact with researchers and patients. JAMA 2003;289(16): 2128–2131.

24. Rogers WJ, Canto JG, Barron HV, et al. Treatment and outcome of myocardial infarction in hospitals with and without invasive capability. J Am Coll Cardiol 2000;35:371–379.

25. Ryan TJ, Anderson JL, Antman EM, et al. ACC/AHA guidelines for the management of patients with acute myocardial infarction: a report of the American College of Cardiology/American Heart Association Task Force on Practice Guidelines (Committee on Management of Acute Myocardial Infarction). J Am Coll Cardiol 1996;28:1328–1428.

26. Lee KL, Woodlief LH, Topol EJ, Weaver WD, Betriu A, Col J, Simoons M, Aylward P, Van de Werf F, Califf RM. Predictors of 30-day mortality in the era of reperfusion for acute myocardial infarction. Results from an international trial of 41,021 patients. GUSTO-I Investigators. Circulation 1995;91(6):1659–1668.

27. Morrow DA, Antman EM, Charlesworth A, et al. TIMI risk score for ST-elevation myocardial infarction: a convenient, bedside, clinical score for risk assessment at presentation: an intravenous nPA for treatment of infarcting myocardium early II trial substudy. Circulation 2000;102(17):2031–2037.

28. Gurwitz JH, Col NF, Avorn J. The exclusion of the elderly and women from clinical trials of acute myocardial infarction. JAMA 1992;268: 1417–1422.

29. Lee PY, Alexander KP, Hammill BG, Pasquali SK, Peterson ED. Representation of elderly persons and women in published randomized trials of acute coronary syndromes JAMA 2001;286(6):708–713.

30. Peterson ED, Lytle BL, Biswas MS, Coombs L. Willingness to participate in cardiac trials. Am J Geriatr Cardiol 2004;13(1):11–15.

31. Cannon CP, Gibson CM, Lambrew CT, Shoultz DA, Levy D, French WJ, Gore JM, Weaver WD, Rogers WJ, Tiefenbrunn AJ. Relationship of symptom-onset-to-balloon time and door-to-balloon time with mortality in patients undergoing angioplasty for acute myocardial infarction. JAMA 2000;283(22):2941–2947.

32. Angeja BG, Gibson CM, Chin R, et al. Participants in the National Registry of Myocardial Infarction 2–3. Predictors of door-to-balloon delay in primary angioplasty. Am J Cardiol 2002;89(10):1156–1161.

33. Topol EJ, Kereiakes DJ. Regionalization of care for acute ischemic heart disease: a call for specialized centers. Circulation 2003;107(11): 1463–1466.

34. Waters RE II, Singh KP, Roe MT, et al. Rationale and strategies for implementing community-based transfer protocols for primary percutaneous coronary intervention for acute ST-segment elevation myocardial infarction. J Am Coll Cardiol. In press.

35. Andersen HR, Nielsen TT, Rasmussen K, et al. A comparison of coronary angioplasty with fibrinolytic therapy in acute myocardial infarction. N Engl J Med 2003;349:733–742.

36. Widimsky P, Groch L, Zelizko M, Aschermann M, Bednar F, Suryapranata H. Multicentre randomized trial comparing transport to primary angioplasty vs. immediate thrombolysis vs. combined strategy for patients with acute myocardial infarction presenting to a community

hospital without a catheterization laboratory. Eur Heart J 2000;21: 823–831.

37. Widimsky P, Budesinsky T, Vorac D, et al., for the PRAGUE Study Group Investigators. Long distance transport for primary angioplasty vs. immediate thrombolysis in acute myocardial infarction. Final results of the randomized national multicentre trial—PRAGUE-2. Eur Heart J 2003; 24(1):94–104.

38. Ryan TJ, Antman EM, Brooks NH, Califf RM, Hillis LD, Hiratzka LF, Rapaport E, Riegel B, Russell RO, Smith EE III, Weaver WD. ACC/AHA guidelines for the management of patients with acute myocardial infarction: 1999 update: a report of the American College of Cardiology/ American Heart Association Task Force on Practice Guidelines (Committee on Management of Acute Myocardial Infarction). Available at http://www.acc.org/clinical/guidelines and http://www.americanheart.org. Accessed on January 15, 2004.

39. Grines CL, Westerhausen DR Jr., Grines LL, et al. A randomized trial of transfer for primary angioplasty versus onsite thrombolysis in patients with high-risk myocardial infarction: the Air Primary Angioplasty in Myocardial Infarction study. J Am Coll Cardiol 2002;39: 1713–1719.

40. Liem A, Zijlstra F, Ottervanger JP, Hoorntje JC, Suryapranata H, de Boer MJ, Verheugt FW. High dose heparin as pretreatment for primary angioplasty in acute myocardial infarction: the Heparin in Early Patency (HEAP) randomized trial. J Am Coll Cardiol 2000;35(3): 600–604.

41. Lincoff AM, Bittl JA, Harrington RA, Feit F, Kleiman NS, Jackman JD, Sarembock IJ, Cohen DJ, Spriggs D, Ebrahimi R, Keren G, Carr J, Cohen EA, Betriu A, Desmet W, Kereiakes DJ, Rutsch W, Wilcox RG, de Feyter PJ, Vahanian A, Topol EJ; REPLACE-2 Investigators. Bivalirudin and provisional glycoprotein IIb/IIIa blockade compared with heparin and planned glycoprotein IIb/IIIa blockade during percutaneous coronary intervention: REPLACE-2 randomized trial. JAMA 2003;289(13):1638.

42. Karagounis L, Ipsen SK, Jessop MR, Gilmore KM, Valenti DA, Clawson JJ, Teichman S, Anderson JL. Impact of field-transmitted electrocardiography on time to in-hospital thrombolytic therapy in acute myocardial infarction. Am J Cardiol 1990;66(10):786–791.

43. Weaver WD, Eisenberg MS, Martin JS, Litwin PE, Shaeffer SM, Ho MT, Kudenchuk P, Hallstrom AP, Cerqueira MD, Copass MK, et al. Myocardial Infarction Triage and Intervention Project—phase I: patient characteristics and feasibility of prehospital initiation of thrombolytic therapy. J Am Coll Cardiol 1990;15(5):925–931.

44. Canto JG, Rogers WJ, Bowlby LJ, French WJ, Pearce DJ, Weaver WD. The prehospital electrocardiogram in acute myocardial infarction: is its full potential being realized? National Registry of Myocardial Infarction 2 Investigators. J Am Coll Cardiol 1997;29(3):498–505.

45. Morrison LJ, Verbeek PR, McDonald AC, Sawadsky BV, Cook DJ. Mortality and prehospital thrombolysis for acute myocardial infarction: a meta-analysis. JAMA 2000;283(20):2686–2692.

46. Wallentin L, Goldstein P, Armstrong PW, Granger CB, Adgey AA, Arntz HR, Bogaerts K, Danays T, Lindahl B, Makijarvi M, Verheugt F, Van de Werf F. Efficacy and safety of tenecteplase in combination with the low-molecular-weight heparin enoxaparin or unfractionated heparin in the prehospital setting: the Assessment of the Safety and Efficacy of a New Thrombolytic Regimen (ASSENT)-3 PLUS randomized trial in acute myocardial infarction. Circulation 2003;108(2): 135–142.

47. Jacobs AK. Primary angioplasty for acute myocardial infarction—is it worth the wait? N Engl J Med 2003;349(8):798–800.

9

Considerations in Reperfusion Therapy of Elderly Patients with ST Elevation Acute Myocardial Infarction

EDWARD L. PORTNAY

Yale University School of Medicine
New Haven, Connecticut, U.S.A.

ALAN K. BERGER

University of Minnesota
Minneapolis, Minnesota, U.S.A.

HARLAN M. KRUMHOLZ

Yale University School of Medicine
and Yale–New Haven Hospital
New Haven, Connecticut, U.S.A.

I. INTRODUCTION

Although the therapeutic benefit of coronary reperfusion—fibrinolytic therapy and primary percutaneous coronary intervention (PCI)—for the treatment of acute ST elevation myocardial infarction (STEMI) in younger patients is well established, there remains considerable debate over the appropriate choice of a reperfusion strategy for elderly patients.

The difficulty in choosing the optimum reperfusion strategy stems from the uncertainty surrounding the data on the efficacy of fibrinolytic therapy in the elderly. Complicating the choice of a strategy for the elderly is the increased risk of bleeding associated with fibrinolytic therapy. Although the data for safety and efficacy for primary PCI are more convincing, primary PCI is not widely available as a reperfusion option (1).

This chapter will first review the data on the efficacy of fibrinolytic therapy among elderly patients. We will define the risk of major hemorrhagic complications associated with fibrinolytic therapy and explain how the available data can be used to help individualize the risk for a given elderly patient. We will also show how, even in eligible patients, there are considerable variations of care across ages, with the elderly receiving fibrinolytic therapy less frequently than younger patients. Finally, we will review the data on the use of primary PCI in elderly patients with STEMI.

II. FIBRINOLYTIC THERAPY

A. Evidence of Efficacy from Randomized Clinical Trials

The difficulty in analyzing data from randomized clinical trials (RCTs) is that no RCT of fibrinolytic therapy focusing specifically on the elderly has ever been completed. The Thrombolytic Therapy in an Older Patient Population (TTOP) trial was designed to study patients >75 years of age presenting with STEMI, randomized to tissue plasminogen activator (t-PA) or placebo (2). This study was the only RCT of fibrinolytic therapy that enrolled only elderly patients. It was discontinued early due to low enrollment. Therefore, all evidence of the treatment in the elderly from RCTs has been obtained from either subgroup analyses of the larger trials or meta-analyses of these studies. In RCTs, study populations have been skewed toward enrolling younger patients. More than 60% of the RCTs excluded patients >75 years of age, and of those that included the elderly, only 10% of the study cohort was composed of those >70 years of age (3). The large RCTs also included all patients with suspicion for acute myocardial infarction (AMI), making it difficult to draw definitive conclusions as to the effectiveness in the setting of confirmed STEMI.

The initial mega-trials of fibrinolytic therapy suggested a benefit in the treatment of the elderly. The Second International Study of Infarct Survival (ISIS-2) randomized 17,187 patients to streptokinase vs. placebo (4). Of these, 3010 patients were 70–79 years of age and 401 patients were ≥80 years of age. Compared with an absolute risk reduction (ARR) of 1.6% (or the number needed to treat to prevent a death, NNT, of 63) in those <60 years of age, there was a 1.9% ARR in those 70–79 years of age and a 14.1% ARR in those ≥80 years of age (NNT = 53 and 7, respectively) (5). Although these reductions in mortality did not reach statistical significance and those ≥80 years of age represented a highly selected population, these data demonstrated that fibrinolytic therapy may be as effective in the elderly as it is in younger patients. In the Gruppo Italiano per lo Studio della Streptochinasi nell'Infarto Miocardico (GISSI-1) trial, which included 11,712 patients randomized to streptokinase or placebo, 10.3% of the study subjects were ≥75 years of age (6). Patients treated with streptokinase had a 4.2% ARR (NNT = 24) in 21-day mortality. Despite the fact that this risk reduction was of greater magnitude than in patients < 65 years of age (ARR 2%, NNT = 50), the reduction did not reach statistical significance secondary to the small size of the elderly cohort.

In a decision analysis based on GISSI and ISIS-2, Krumholz et al. evaluated the choice to administer fibrinolytic therapy to patients ≥75 years of age (7). The short-term mortality rate for patients in this age group was estimated by pooling the results of GISSI and ISIS-2 (29%). The overall analysis and several sensitivity analyses demonstrated that the decision favored treatment even with low estimates of percent reduction in mortality or with high risks of major bleeding. A cost-effectiveness analysis also revealed that use of fibrinolytic therapy was economically very attractive. Overall, the results demonstrated that the high risk associated with elderly STEMI patients means that any therapy that produces even a modest relative reduction in risk can save many lives. Thus, the NNT for elderly patients is relatively small. Moreover, the high underlying risk of the STEMI means that the risk of the therapy is easily offset by the benefit until the risk becomes very high (>4%).

In 1994, the benefit of fibrinolytic therapy in the treatment of the elderly was brought into question by the Fibrinolytic Therapy Trialists' (FTT) Collaborative Group (3). This meta-analysis included nine fibrinolytic trials incorporating over 58,600 patients. Of these patients, 17,000 were 65–74 years of age and 5754 were ≥75 years of age. This analysis revealed that the benefit of fibrinolytic therapy diminished with advancing age: relative risk reduction (RRR) of death associated with fibrinolytic therapy was 22% in patients <55 years of age, 19% in patients 55–64 years of age, 16% in patients 65–74 years of age and only 4% in patients ≥75 years of age. However, while the relative effectiveness of fibrinolytic therapy diminished with advancing age, the 4% RRR translated into a 1% ARR, or NNT = 100, still a clinically important difference and similar to the 1.2% ARR in patients <55 years of age. Therefore, even small relative reductions in risk can be important when applied to groups with increased risk.

Of the nine trials included in the FTT meta-analysis, Late Assessment of Thrombolytic Efficacy (LATE) and Estudio Multicéntrico Estreptoquinasa Repúblicas de América del Sur (EMERAS) enrolled only patients who presented ≥6 hours after the onset of chest pain (8,9). Both of these studies demonstrated minimal benefit from fibrinolytic therapy as compared to the impressive reductions seen in GISSI and ISIS-2 (8.9% mortality in the t-PA group vs. 10.3% mortality in the control group in LATE and no benefit of streptokinase over control in patients presenting >12 hours after symptom onset in EMERAS). The inclusion of these two trials diluted the effects of fibrinolytic therapy in the FTT analysis. Furthermore, in the prematurely terminated APSAC Intervention Mortality Study (AIMS), only 3 of the total 502 patients were >70 years of age, raising concerns about the ability of the FTT to extrapolate these results to elderly patients (10).

Since the original publication of the FTT, White reported unpublished data from the FTT that shows a more sustained benefit in the elderly (11). In contrast to the initial FTT analysis that included patients with factors associated with both reduced benefit and increased risk of fibrinolytic therapy (i.e., patients presenting >12 hours after the onset of symptoms as well as individuals showing ST depression or T wave inversions), the new analysis focused on elderly patients who were "ideal candidates" for fibrinolytic therapy: patients ≥75 years of age presenting within 12 hours of symptom onset with ST elevation or left bundle branch block. When only these patients were analyzed, the RRR of death associated with fibrinolytic therapy was 15%, with an ARR of 3.4% (NNT = 29). This is similar to the NNT = 40 in patients 65–74 years of age although greater than NNT = 16 in patients <55 years of age. This magnitude of difference is clearly clinically important and more consistent with the findings of ISIS-2 and GISSI-1.

B. Observational Studies of Fibrinolytic Efficacy among the Elderly

RCTs produced data that raised questions about the relative benefit of fibrinolytic therapy in the elderly—diminished RRRs and clinically important but not statistically significant ARRs. Similarly, one observational study showed that fibrinolytic therapy may be associated with increased harm, whereas two others have shown long-term mortality benefit of fibrinolytic therapy when applied in "real-world" situations. The study that has received the most attention is the Thiemann et al. analysis of the Cooperative Cardiovascular Project (CCP) (12). The CCP was developed by the Centers for Medicare and Medicaid Services (formerly called the Health Care Financing Administration) as an initiative to improve the quality of care of Medicare beneficiaries with AMI. In this analysis, exclusions included patients <65 years of age, patients at hospitals with on-site angioplasty, patients who presented >12 hours after symptom onset, patients with left bundle branch block, patients with absolute contraindications to fibrinolytic therapy, and patients who did not receive aspirin or heparin therapy. Although patients 65–75 years of age treated with fibrinolytic therapy had a lower crude mortality rate and adjusted hazard ratio (HR) for 30-day mortality (6.8% vs. 9.8%; HR 0.76; 95% CI 0.61–0.95), patients 76–86 years of age had increased mortality at 30 days (18.0% vs. 15.4%; HR 1.29; 95% CI 1.06–1.58). This alarming study was the first observational study or randomized trial to pose the possibility that the utilization of fibrinolytic therapy in the elderly subgroup might not only have diminished efficacy but actually conferred an increased risk of death.

In contrast, Berger et al. (13) published a separate analysis from the same database, which expanded on the Thiemann analysis. In addition to key differences in patient selection between the two CCP analyses described below, Berger et al. included long-term follow-up outcomes. This analysis not only compared fibrinolytic therapy to no reperfusion therapy but also included a comparison with primary PCI. As opposed to the Thiemann analysis, Berger et al. created an "ideal" subgroup that excluded patients with reperfusion >6 hours from symptom onset and patients with either absolute or relative contraindications to fibrinolysis: these contraindications included prior internal bleeding; recent trauma, surgery, or cardiopulmonary resuscitation; any prior stroke; uncontrolled hypertension; patient or physician refusal of fibrinolytic therapy; and current use of warfarin with an International Normalized Ratio > 2.0. In this analysis, crude 30-day mortality rates revealed a benefit of fibrinolytic therapy both in the patients with no absolute contraindications (20.6% vs. 13.5%; $p = 0.001$) and for the "ideal" patients (14.8% vs. 10.6%; $p = 0.001$). Although the adjusted 30-day mortality model for the "ideal" patients revealed no significant benefit with fibrinolytic therapy at 30 days (OR 1.05; 95% CI 0.93–1.19), fibrinolytic therapy was associated with lower mortality at one year (OR 0.84; CI 0.79–0.89). This benefit was consistent across all ages, even in those ≥85 years of age. Compared with the harm associated with fibrinolytic therapy shown by Thiemann et al., Berger et al.'s stricter patient selection revealed no short-term harm and a significant long-term mortality benefit associated with fibrinolytic therapy in the elderly.

Further data demonstrating the long-term benefit of fibrinolytic therapy were reported by Stenestrand et al. (14). This registry enrolled every patient admitted to the coronary care unit of 64 Swedish hospitals between 1995 and 1999. Of the 50,779 admissions, 19,052 were a first-recorded admission for STEMI and 6891 patients ≥75 years of age received either fibrinolytic therapy or no reperfusion. In contrast to the Berger et al. analysis, fibrinolytic therapy was associated with both reductions in adjusted 30-day mortality (23% vs. 26%; $p = 0.02$) and adjusted one-year mortality (32% vs. 36%; $p = 0.001$).

C. Selection of Fibrinolytic Agent

Since the initial fibrinolytic trials, there have been multiple studies comparing thrombolytic agents. To date, no study has specifically compared the efficacy and safety profile of one individual fibrinolytic agent with another for the elderly subgroup of patients. However, several comparative studies have enrolled a sufficient number of patients to permit subgroup analyses of the elderly. The Global Utilization of Streptokinase and Tissue Plasminogen Activator for Occluded Coronary Arteries (GUSTO)-1 trial was conceived to test the hypothesis that t-PA (a fibrin-specific agent that leads to early and more complete patency rates of the infarct-related artery) would be superior to streptokinase in survival outcomes (15). Of the 41,021 patients enrolled in the study, 2358 patients >75 years of age were randomized to streptokinase and 1297 patients >75 years of age were randomized to t-PA. The trial revealed that there was a lower rate of death or disabling stroke for all age groups treated with t-PA compared with streptokinase, except for those >85 years of age, in whom streptokinase produced a lower rate of death or disabling stroke. There were small increases in the absolute risk of hemorrhagic stroke with t-PA use in patients 65–74 and 75–84 years of age (1.14% vs. 0.55%; OR 2.1; 95% CI 1.13–3.88; and 2.14% vs. 1.24%; OR 1.74; 95% CI 0.89–3.41, respectively). These complications were offset by the relatively large 2% ARR of death in older patients treated with t-PA as compared to streptokinase (8.3% vs. 10.4%; OR 0.77; 95% CI 0.64–0.93; and 18.2% vs. 20.2%, OR 0.88; 95% CI 0.71–1.08, respectively, for the two age groups). Nevertheless, given the small sample size of the elderly subgroups, these benefits were not statistically significant.

In the Assessment of the Safety and Efficacy of a New Thrombolytic Regimen (ASSENT)-2 trial, tenecteplase (TNK) was compared with t-PA (16). Although older age was an independent risk factor for major bleeding, there was a statistically nonsignificant 2% absolute difference in 30-day mortality between the two fibrinolytic agents in those more than 75 years of age (17.4% with TNK and 19.3% with t-PA; RR 0.9; CI 0.75–1.08). GUSTO-III was a multinational study that randomized 15,059 patients, 13.5% of whom were older than 75 years. In this large trial, reteplase was compared with t-PA. There was no difference between reteplase and t-PA in either 30-day or 1-year mortality or in the rates of stroke among the total study cohort and among those ≤75 years of age and those >75 years of age (17,18). Thus, to date, t-PA, reteplase, and TNK appear to have similar outcomes for elderly patients treated with fibrinolytic therapy, whereas streptokinase appears inferior with respect to mortality.

D. Combined Fibrinolytic and Glycoprotein IIbIIIa Inhibitor Therapy

Recent trials have explored the combination of fibrinolytic agents with glycoprotein IIbIIIa (GP IIbIIIa) inhibitors and low molecular weight heparins (LMWH) to further advance the benefits of fibrinolytic therapy alone. Researchers hypothesized that the addition of GP IIbIIIa inhibitors to fibrinolytic therapy at lower dosages would lead to improved reperfusion as well as fewer hemorrhagic complications. Both the ASSENT-3 and GUSTO-V trials tested this approach in large-scale RCTs (19,20). In the GUSTO-V trial, 16,588 patients were randomly assigned standard-dose reteplase versus half-dose reteplase combined with full-dose abciximab. While there was a trend toward benefit of the combination therapy in those ≤75 years of age, there was a trend toward increased mortality among elderly patients treated with combination therapy. There was also a trend toward an increase in intracranial hemorrhage in patients >75 years of age treated with combination therapy versus reteplase alone (OR 1.91; CI 0.95–3.94). There was a significant interaction between treatment and older age for intracranial hemorrhage.

In ASSENT-3, 6095 patients were randomized to one of three regimens: full-dose TNK and enoxaparin, half-dose TNK with weight-adjusted low-dose unfractionated heparin and a 12-hour infusion of abciximab, or full-dose TNK with weight-adjusted unfractionated heparin. Although there was a benefit for combination therapy seen in patients ≤75 years of age, for those >75 years of age there was no significant difference between the three treatment arms in terms of the combined safety endpoint (death at 30 days, in-hospital reinfarction or refractory ischemia, intracranial hemorrhage (ICH), or major bleeding).

There was a trend toward increased 30-day mortality among patients treated with TNK and abciximab compared with those treated with TNK and unfractionated heparin or TNK and LMWH. Given these findings, the ASSENT-3 authors concluded that "caution should be exercised regarding the use of conjunctive therapy with abciximab in elderly patients with an AMI treated with a fibrinolytic agent."

Further caution regarding the use of more powerful conjunctive antithrombotic or antiplatelet therapies in the elderly was demonstrated in the subsequent ASSENT-3 PLUS trial (21). This trial randomized 1639 patients with STEMI to prehospital fibrinolysis with either unfractionated heparin or enoxaparin. While enoxaparin reduced the risk of reinfarction as compared to unfractionated heparin, it came at the price of significantly increasing the rate of bleeding. The nearly 10-fold increase in intracranial bleeding among elderly patients treated with the combination of enoxaparin and TNK (as opposed to TNK and unfractionated heparin) was a potent reminder of the increased risk for adverse events in elderly patients with STEMI. Given these safety concerns, especially among the elderly, neither glycoprotein IIbIIIa inhibitors nor LMWH has provided sufficient additional efficacy to supplant the standard TNK or reteplase regimens utilized with unfractionated heparin.

E. Estimating the Risk of Fibrinolytic Therapy in the Elderly

Of all the complications of reperfusion therapy, the risk of ICH with fibrinolytic therapy is the most feared. In multiple RCTs and observational studies, age has been reported to be strongly associated with bleeding complications (3,22–24). In the GUSTO-1 trial (22), age was the most powerful predictor of hemorrhagic stroke with increased risk with advancing age. While the risk in those <65 years of age was 0.8%, this increased to 3.4% in those 75–84 years of age. Data from observational studies have shown similar rates of stroke to those seen in clinical trials. In the National Registry of Myocardial Infarction (NRMI) 2 registry, Gurwitz et al. found that the incidence of ICH increased with age (25). While the incidence of ICH was 0.4% in those <65 years of age, the incidence increased to 1.23% in those 65–74 years of age and 2.13% in those ≥75 years of age. In multivariate analysis, age was the most powerful predictor of ICH. Compared with those <65 years of age, patients aged 65–74 years had an almost threefold odd increase of ICH (OR 2.71, 2.18–3.37) and patients ≥75 years of age had an almost 4.5-fold odds increase in risk of ICH (OR 4.34, 3.45–5.45).

Although all fibrinolytic agents are associated with an increased risk of ICH, data suggest that this risk in the elderly is higher with t-PA compared with streptokinase. In GUSTO-1, t-PA was compared with streptokinase and associated with an increase in the absolute risk of hemorrhagic stroke in patients 65–74 years of age and 75–84 years of age (1.14% vs. 0.55%; OR 2.1; 95% CI 1.13–3.88; and 2.14% vs. 1.24%; OR 1.74; 95% CI 0.89–3.41, respectively) (15). Although ASSENT-2 failed to report on the rate of ICH by age for TNK versus t-PA (16), GUSTO III did report an increased trend toward ICH with reteplase versus t-PA in patients >75 years of age (2.5% vs. 1.7%) (17). As previously mentioned, combination therapy of either reteplase or TNK with a GP IIbIIIa inhibitor was associated with increased risk of ICH (19,20). Similarly, combining TNK with enoxaparin significantly increased the risk of intracranial bleeding (21). Thus, there has been limited progress in reducing the rate of intracranial bleeding among elderly patients utilizing more recent fibrinolytic regimens.

While age is associated with increased risk of bleeding, it is only one of several key factors that must be considered in estimating an individual patient's risk of ICH. Brass et al. examined the risk of hemorrhagic stroke in Medicare patients presenting with AMI (26). Overall, the rate of ICH was 1.5%. Certain characteristics—age ≥75 years, female, black race, prior stroke, elevated blood pressure, t-PA, excessive anticoagulation, and low body weight—were all independently associated with increased risk of ICH. Brass et al. then developed a risk stratification scale based on the independent factors associated with ICH. In patients with ≥5 of the above factors, the rate of ICH was as high as 4.11% (Tables 9.1 and 9.2). This tool enables physicians to estimate an individual's risk with the use of these easily identified factors. With an understanding of an individual's risk, physicians and their patients can decide to utilize fibrinolytic therapy given the high

Table 9.1 Factors Associated with Intracranial Hemorrhage Based on Multiple Logistic Regression

Factor	Adjusted odds ratio	95% confidence interval	p-value
Age ≥ 75 y	1.57	1.30–1.90	0.0001
Black	1.63	1.12–2.36	0.0099
Female	1.39	1.15–1.68	0.0006
Prior stroke	1.49	1.11–2.01	0.0089
Systolic BP ≥ 160 mmHg	1.81	1.50–2.19	0.0001
Weight below median value	1.47	1.22–1.78	0.0001
t-PA use (vs. other thrombolytic agent)	1.57	1.23–2.00	0.0003

Adjusted odds ratios were derived from a multiple logistic regression analysis in which each odds ratio was adjusted for all other factors listed. An odds ratio higher than 1 indicates that patients with the characteristic have a higher likelihood of having an intracranial hemorrhage than those without the characteristic.
Source: Ref. 26.

Table 9.2 Risk of Hemorrhagic Stroke Using the Seven Factors from Table 9.1

Number of factors	n^a	Percent	Hemorrhagic stroke (%)	Adjusted odds ratio	95% confidence interval
0 or 1	6,721	21.3	0.71	1.00	
2	10,533	33.3	1.01	1.36	0.98–1.91
3	9,061	28.7	1.64	2.23	1.63–3.10
4	4,256	13.5	2.51	3.44	2.47–4.85
≥5	1,032	3.3	4.07	5.66	3.72–8.54

[a] Missing data on 129 cases.
Source: Ref. 26.

mortality rate in the elderly with an acceptable risk for ICH, or select an alternative reperfusion strategy in patients at especially high risk.

F. Patterns of Use of Fibrinolytic Therapy in the Elderly

Multiple observational studies have shown that the likelihood of receiving fibrinolytic therapy decreases with increasing age (27–30). This pattern is in part related to the decrease in the eligibility rates for fibrinolytic therapy among the elderly. Evidence of this trend comes from the Multicenter Chest Pain Study, an analysis of 12,140 patients presenting to three university and four community emergency departments with the chief complaint of chest pain (27). Of the 1584 patients with a diagnosed AMI, 746 were >65 years of age. The proportion of patients with ideal eligibility for fibrinolytic therapy (patients arriving within 6 hours of the onset of pain with ST segment elevation or pathological Q-waves not known to be old) decreased from 34% in patients <65 years of age to 18% for those ≥75 years of age.

However, the disproportionately low rate of fibrinolytic therapy use in the elderly is not fully explained by the lower rates of eligibility. Even among eligible elderly patients, the rates of fibrinolytic therapy use are lower than in younger eligible patients. Krumholz et al. examined a cohort of 3093 patients ≥65 years of age with a discharge diagnosis of AMI covered by Medicare from May 1992 to May 1993 in Connecticut (29). Among the beneficiaries eligible for fibrinolytic therapy, increasing age was still associated with decreasing use of fibrinolytic therapy: 58.5% in patients 65–74 years of age, 37.7% in patients 75–84 years of age, and 16.4% in patients ≥85 years of age. This pattern of decreasing use of fibrinolytic therapy, even among eligible elderly patients, was also shown in the Worcester Heart Attack Study (30). This registry comprised 3824 patients admitted to hospitals in the Worcester, Massachusetts, area with a confirmed AMI from 1986 through 1993. Among eligible patients, the rate of fibrinolytic therapy use was lower in the elderly. Only 31% of those >74 years of age received fibrinolytic therapy compared with 68% of those <55 years of age. This same pattern was also shown to exist by Barron et al. from NRMI-2 (31), who reported that almost one third of all non-transferred patients were eligible for reperfusion therapy. Of those eligible, 24% were not given this therapy. The elderly, along with women, patients without chest pain on admission, and those patients with the highest risk for in-hospital mortality were least likely to receive reperfusion therapy. Thus, there appear to be multiple barriers to broad utilization of a fibrinolytic therapy approach among elderly patients with STEMI.

III. PRIMARY PERCUTANEOUS CORONARY INTERVENTION

Primary PCI has been shown to be safe and effective as a reperfusion strategy in the elderly (31–33). Although some of the trials comparing primary PCI with fibrinolytic therapy have excluded elderly patients, two landmark studies—Primary Angioplasty in Myocardial Infarction (PAMI) and GUSTO-2b—enrolled sufficient numbers of elderly patients to examine the treatment effect of primary PCI in this group (31,33). Overall, the PAMI trial showed that primary PCI compared with fibrinolytic therapy led to a reduction in the rate of nonfatal reinfarction and death from 12% (95% CI 7.5–16.5) to 5.1% (95% CI 2.1–8.1) ($p = 0.02$). In those considered "not low risk," which included all patients >70 years of age, there was a >8% ARR of death from 10.4% (4.6–16.2%) to 2.0% (0–4.7%) ($p = 0.01$), NNT = 12.5. In the GUSTO 2b trial, 1138 patients were randomized to t-PA vs. angioplasty. In the entire cohort, 30-day mortality was reduced from 7% to 5.7% in patients treated with angioplasty vs. t-PA (OR 0.8; 95% CI 0.49–1.3). Among patients >70 years of age (26% of the total cohort), there was a strong trend favoring PCI over t-PA. The relatively small percentage of elderly patients in this trial may explain why the benefit of PCI did not reach statistical significance.

Of the 23 trials comparing fibrinolytic therapy to primary PCI, only one has exclusively enrolled elderly patients (32,34). In this single center study from the Netherlands, 87 patients ≥76 years of age were randomized to streptokinase ($n = 41$) versus primary angioplasty ($n = 46$). Patients were excluded if they had contraindications for fibrinolytic therapy or if they presented >6 hours after symptom onset. The median age was 80 in the angioplasty arm and 81 in the t-PA arm. The composite endpoint of death, recurrent AMI, and stroke at 30 days was 9% in the angioplasty arm and 29% in the streptokinase arm (RR 4.3; 95% CI 1.2–20.0). Despite the small size of this study, there were significant reductions in in-hospital mortality (7% vs. 20%; $p = 0.07$; RR for streptokinase not provided), 30-day mortality (7% vs. 22%; $p = 0.04$; RR for streptokinase 4.0; 95% CI 0.9–24.6), and 1-year mortality (11% vs. 29%; $p = 0.03$; RR for streptokinase 3.4; 95% CI 1.0–13.5). This study was halted prematurely given the magnitude of benefit of primary angioplasty vs. streptokinase on the incidence of 30-day mortality and the combined endpoint at 30 days.

Numerous observational studies have confirmed the treatment benefit seen in the above RCTs of primary PCI as a reperfusion strategy in the elderly. In the previously mentioned analysis of the CCP, Berger et al. found primary PCI compared with no reperfusion was associated with significant reductions in both 30-day and 1-year mortality among patients without absolute contraindications for fibrinolytic therapy (13). Among the "ideal" patient subgroup, primary PCI yielded reductions in adjusted mortality rates at 30 days and at 1 year compared with no therapy (OR 0.78, 95% CI 0.58–1.05; and OR 0.63, 95% CI 0.49–0.84). However, since this analysis used no reperfusion therapy as the comparison group, primary PCI and fibrinolytic therapy were not directly compared.

In a separate analysis of the CCP, Berger et al. compared primary PCI directly to fibrinolytic therapy (36). The outcomes of 18,645 patients who received fibrinolytic therapy were compared with 2038 patients who received primary PCI. This cohort was composed of patients >65 years of age, not in cardiogenic shock, within 12 hours from symptom onset and with no contraindications to fibrinolytic therapy. Among the entire cohort, primary PCI resulted in lower crude and adjusted rates of 30-day and 1-year mortality. The benefit of PCI persisted even in those >75 years of age.

The efficacy of primary PCI was also shown by Zahn et al. in a pooled analysis of the Maximal Individual Therapy in Acute Myocardial Infarction (MITRA) and the Myocardial Infarction Registry (MIR) Study Groups (37). The MITRA (1994–1997) and MIR (1996–1998) registries were both German, prospective, multicenter, observational studies of the treatment of patients with AMI. Fifty-four hospitals participated in the MITRA study. The MIR study was a nationwide registry that included a total of 217 hospitals (mainly community hospitals). In this analysis of more than 9000 fibrinolytic-eligible patients, PCI was consistently associated with a reduction of in-hospital mortality across all ages, with a roughly 40% reduction in the risk of in-hospital mortality in those ≥75 years. As absolute mortality increased, there was an increasing benefit of PCI over fibrinolytic therapy.

Despite these impressive results, not all elderly patients with STEMI have been shown to benefit from primary PCI. Data from the Should We Emergently Revascularize Occluded Coronaries for Cardiogenic Shock (SHOCK) trial revealed that although patients < 75 years of age presenting in cardiogenic shock benefited from early invasive revascularization compared with medical therapy, those ≥75 years of age experienced greater mortality at both 30 days and 6 months (38). In a separate report on the one-year follow-up, patients >75 years of age still derived no benefit from early revascularization, compared with the benefit in younger patients (39). In contrast to the above trial, an analysis of the SHOCK registry (a large, prospective multicenter registry of patients with cardiogenic shock not enrolled in the SHOCK trial) revealed early revascularization to be effective for elderly patients in SHOCK (40). Compared with the very limited sample of 56 elderly patients in the trial, 32% of the registry's 877 patients were ≥75 years of age. In the registry, the rate of in-hospital mortality in the early- vs. late- or no-revascularization group was 48% vs. 81% ($p = 0.0003$). After covariate-adjusted modeling, early revascularization remained independently associated with a mortality benefit. Two other registries—the Worcester Heart Attack Study and the Northern New England Cardiovascular Group—have similarly shown improving outcomes for selected elderly shock patients managed with early coronary revascularization (41,42). One explanation for the difference in results between the RCT and registry studies may be the selection of elderly patients with a lack of comorbidities frequently associated with old age.

IV. CONCLUSIONS

Despite decades of study, uncertainty still remains about the optimal treatment strategy for the elderly patient with STEMI. There is mounting evidence that primary PCI is a safe and efficacious means of reperfusion and is superior to fibrinolytic therapy. Therefore, primary PCI, if available, should probably be the treatment of choice in the elderly patient with STEMI. However, primary PCI is not readily available as a reperfusion modality at many of the institutions that admit patients with STEMI. Thus, fibrinolytic therapy may be the only reperfusion strategy from which to choose. Although the data from RCTs show decreasing relative risk reductions as age increases, fibrinolytic therapy still yields clinically significant absolute reductions in events. Furthermore, data from observational studies have shown long-term mortality benefits from fibrinolytic therapy. Therefore, fibrinolytic therapy is an effective means of improving outcomes in the elderly. Although the rates of eligibility for fibrinolytic therapy decrease with advancing age, those that are eligible should be offered this therapy. Nevertheless, both RCTs and observational studies have shown that despite the effectiveness of both strategies, these treatment effects are not universally provided to all elderly patients. The best approach is to take into account individual patients' risk of complications, their expected benefit, and their treatment goals when making the decision about this approach.

REFERENCES

1. Rogers WJ, Canto JG, Barron HV, Boscarino JA, Shoultz DA, Every NR. Treatment and outcome of myocardial infarction in hospitals with and without invasive capability. Investigators in the National Registry of Myocardial Infarction. J Am Coll Cardiol 2000;35:371–379.

2. Feit F, Breed J, Anderson JL. A randomized, placebo-controlled trial of tissue plasminogen activator in elderly patients with acute myocardial infarction (abstr). Circulation 1991;82.

3. Indications for fibrinolytic therapy in suspected acute myocardial infarction: collaborative overview of early mortality and major morbidity results from all randomised trials of more than 1000 patients. Fibrinolytic Therapy Trialists' (FTT) Collaborative Group. Lancet 1994;343: 311–322.

4. Randomised trial of intravenous streptokinase, oral aspirin, both, or neither among 17,187 cases of suspected acute myocardial infarction: ISIS-2. ISIS-2 (Second International Study of Infarct Survival) Collaborative Group. Lancet 1988;2:349–360.

5. Rich MW. Thrombolytic therapy is indicated for patients over 75 years of age with ST-elevation acute myocardial infarction: protagonist viewpoint. Am J Geriatr Cardiol 2003;12:344–347.

6. Effectiveness of intravenous thrombolytic treatment in acute myocardial infarction. Gruppo Italiano per lo Studio della Streptochinasi nell'Infarto Miocardico (GISSI). Lancet 1986;1:397–402.

7. Krumholz HM, Pasternak RC, Weinstein MC, Friesinger GC, Ridker PM, Tosteson AN, Goldman L. Cost effectiveness of thrombolytic therapy with streptokinase in elderly patients with suspected acute myocardial infarction. N Engl J Med 1992;327:7–13.

8. Randomised trial of late thrombolysis in patients with suspected acute myocardial infarction. EMERAS (Estudio Multicéntrico Estreptoquinasa Repúblicas de América del Sur) Collaborative Group. Lancet 1993;342:767–772.

9. Late Assessment of Thrombolytic Efficacy (LATE) study with alteplase 6–24 hours after onset of acute myocardial infarction. Lancet 1993;342: 759–766.

10. Effect of intravenous APSAC on mortality after acute myocardial infarction: preliminary report of a placebo-controlled clinical trial. AIMS Trial Study Group. Lancet 1988;1:545–549.

11. White HD. Thrombolytic therapy in the elderly. Lancet 2000;356: 2028–2030.

12. Thiemann DR, Coresh J, Schulman SP, Gerstenblith G, Oetgen WJ, Powe NR. Lack of benefit for intravenous thrombolysis in patients with myocardial infarction who are older than 75 years. Circulation 2000; 101:2239–2246.

13. Berger AK, Radford MJ, Wang Y, Krumholz HM. Thrombolytic therapy in older patients. J Am Coll Cardiol 2000;36:366–374.

14. Stenestrand U, Wallentin L. Fibrinolytic therapy in patients 75 years and older with ST-segment-elevation myocardial infarction: one-year follow-up of a large prospective cohort. Arch Intern Med 2003;163: 965–971.

15. An international randomized trial comparing four thrombolytic strategies for acute myocardial infarction. The GUSTO Investigators. N Engl J Med 1993;329:673–682.

16. Single-bolus tenecteplase compared with front-loaded alteplase in acute myocardial infarction: the ASSENT-2 double-blind randomised

trial. Assessment of the Safety and Efficacy of a New Thrombolytic Investigators. Lancet 1999;354:716–722.

17. A comparison of reteplase with alteplase for acute myocardial infarction. The Global Use of Strategies to Open Occluded Coronary Arteries (GUSTO III) Investigators. N Engl J Med 1997;337:1118–1123.

18. Topol EJ, Ohman EM, Armstrong PW, Wilcox R, Skene AM, Aylward P, Simes J, Dalby A, Betriu A, Bode C, White HD, Hochman JS, Emanuelson H, Vahanian A, Sapp S, Stebbins A, Moliterno DT, Califf RM. Survival outcomes 1 year after reperfusion therapy with either alteplase or reteplase for acute myocardial infarction: results from the Global Utilization of Streptokinase and t-PA for Occluded Coronary Arteries (GUSTO) III Trial. Circulation 2000;102:1761–1765.

19. Topol EJ. Reperfusion therapy for acute myocardial infarction with fibrinolytic therapy or combination reduced fibrinolytic therapy and platelet glycoprotein IIb/IIIa inhibition: the GUSTO V randomised trial. Lancet 2001;357:1905–1914.

20. Efficacy and safety of tenecteplase in combination with enoxaparin, abciximab, or unfractionated heparin: the ASSENT-3 randomised trial in acute myocardial infarction. Lancet 2001;358:605–613.

21. Wallentin L, Goldstein P, Armstrong PW, Granger CB, Adgey AA, Arntz H.R, Bogaerts K, Danays T, Lindahl B, Makijarvi M, Verheugt F, Van de Werf F. Efficacy and safety of tenecteplase in combination with the low-molecular-weight heparin enoxaparin or unfractionated heparin in the prehospital setting: the Assessment of the Safety and Efficacy of a New Thrombolytic Regimen (ASSENT)-3 PLUS randomized trial in acute myocardial infarction. Circulation 2003;108: 135–142

22. White HD, Barbash GI, Califf RM, Simes RJ, Granger CB, Weaver WD, Kleiman NS, Aylward RP, Gore JM, Vahanian A, Lee KL, Ross AM, Topol EJ. Age and outcome with contemporary thrombolytic therapy. Results from the GUSTO-I trial. Global Utilization of Streptokinase and TPA for Occluded coronary arteries trial. Circulation 1996;94:1826–1833.

23. Gore JM, Granger CB, Simoons ML, Sloan MA, Weaver ND, White HD, Barbash GI, Van de Werf F, Aylward PE, Topol EJ, et al. Stroke after thrombolysis. Mortality and functional outcomes in the GUSTO-I

trial. Global Use of Strategies to Open Occluded Coronary Arteries. Circulation 1995;92:2811–2818.

24. Gebel JM, Sila CA, Sloan MA, Granger CB, Mahaffey KW, Weisenberger J, Green CL, White HD, Gore JM, Weaver WD, Califf RM, Topol EJ. Thrombolysis-related intracranial hemorrhage: a radiographic analysis of 244 cases from the GUSTO-1 trial with clinical correlation. Global Utilization of Streptokinase and Tissue Plasminogen Activator for Occluded Coronary Arteries. Stroke 1998;29:563– 569.

25. Gurwitz JH, Gore JM, Goldberg RJ, Barron HV, Breen T, Rundle AC, Sloan MA, French W, Rogers WJ. Risk for intracranial hemorrhage after tissue plasminogen activator treatment for acute myocardial infarction. Participants in the National Registry of Myocardial Infarction 2. Ann Intern Med 1998;129:597–604.

26. Brass LM, Lichtman JH, Wang Y, Gurwitz JH, Radford MJ, Krumholz HM. Intracranial hemorrhage associated with thrombolytic therapy for elderly patients with acute myocardial infarction: results from the Cooperative Cardiovascular Project. Stroke 2000;31:1802–1811.

27. Krumholz HM, Friesinger GC, Cook EF, Lee TH, Rouan GW, Goldman L. Relationship of age with eligibility for thrombolytic therapy and mortality among patients with suspected acute myocardial infarction. J Am Geriatr Soc 1994;42:127–131.

28. Krumholz HM, Gross CP, Peterson ED, Barron HV, Radford MJ, Parsons LS, Every NR. Is there evidence of implicit exclusion criteria for elderly subjects in randomized trials? Evidence from the GUSTO-1. Am Heart J 2003;146:839–847.

29. Krumholz HM, Murillo JE, Chen J, Vaccarino V, Radford MJ, Ellerbeck EF, Wang Y. Thrombolytic therapy for eligible elderly patients with acute myocardial infarction. JAMA 1997;277:1683–1688.

30. Chandra H, Yarzebski J, Goldberg RJ, Savageau J, Singleton C, Gurwitz JH, Gore JM. Age-related trends (1986–1993) in the use of thrombolytic agents in patients with acute myocardial infarction. The Worcester Heart Attack Study. Arch Intern Med 1997;157:741–746.

31. Barron HV, Rundle A, Gurwitz J, Tiefenbrunn A. Reperfusion therapy for acute myocardial infarction: observations from the National Registry of Myocardial Infarction 2. Cardiol Rev 1999;7:156–160.

32. Grines CL, Browne KF, Marco J, Rothbaum D, Stone DW, O'Keefe J, Overlie P, Donohue B, Chelliah N, Timmis GS, et al. A comparison of immediate angioplasty with thrombolytic therapy for acute myocardial infarction. The Primary Angioplasty in Myocardial Infarction Study Group. N Engl J Med 1993;328:673–679.

33. de Boer M-J, Ottervanger J-P, van't Hof AW, Hoorntje JC, Suryapranata H, Zijlstra F. Zwolle Myocardial Infarction Group. Reperfusion therapy in elderly patients with acute myocardial infarction: a randomized comparison of primary angioplasty and thrombolytic therapy. J Am Coll Cardiol 2002;39:1723–1728.

34. A clinical trial comparing primary coronary angioplasty with tissue plasminogen activator for acute myocardial infarction. The Global Use of Strategies to Open Occluded Coronary Arteries in Acute Coronary Syndromes (GUSTO IIb) Angioplasty Substudy Investigators. N Engl J Med 1997;336:1621–1628.

35. Keeley EC, Boura JA, Grines CL. Primary angioplasty versus intravenous thrombolytic therapy for acute myocardial infarction: a quantitative review of 23 randomised trials. Lancet 2003;361:13–20.

36. Berger AK, Schulman KA, Gersh BJ, Pirzada S, Breall JA, Johnson AE, Every NR. Primary coronary angioplasty vs. thrombolysis for the management of acute myocardial infarction in elderly patients. JAMA 1999;282:341–348.

37. Zahn R, Schiele R, Schneider S, Gitt AK, Wienberger H, Seidl K, Voigtlander T, Gottwik M, Berg G, Altman E, Rosahl W, Senges J. Primary angioplasty versus intravenous thrombolysis in acute myocardial infarction: can we define subgroups of patients benefiting most from primary angioplasty? Results from the pooled data of the Maximal Individual Therapy in Acute Myocardial Infarction Registry and the Myocardial Infarction Registry. J Am Coll Cardiol 2001;37:1827–1835.

38. Hochman JS, Sleeper LA, Webb JG, Sanborn TA, White HD, Talley JD, Buller CE, Jacobs AK, Slater JN, Col J, McKinlay SM, LeJemtel TH. Early revascularization in acute myocardial infarction complicated by cardiogenic shock. SHOCK Investigators. Should we emergently revascularize occluded coronaries for cardiogenic shock? N Engl J Med 1999;341:625–634.

39. SHOCK Investigators. One-year survival following early revascularization for cardiogenic shock. JAMA 2001;285:190–192.

40. Dzavik V, Sleeper LA, Cocke TP, Moscucci M, Saucedo J, Hosat S, Jiang X, Slater J, LeJemtel TH, Hochman JS. Early revascularization is associated with improved survival in elderly patients with acute myocardial infarction complicated by cardiogenic shock: a report from the SHOCK Trial Registry. Eur Heart J 2003;24:828–837.

41. Dauerman HL, Goldberg RJ, Malinski M, Yarzebski J, Lessard D, Gore JM. Outcomes and early revascularization for elderly patients with acute myocardial infarction complicated by cardiogenic shock: a population based perspective. Am J Cardiol 2001;87:844–848.

42. Dauerman HL, Ryan TJ, Malenka DM, et al. Outcomes of percutaneous coronary intervention among elderly patients in cardiogenic shock: a multi-center, decade long experience. J Inv Cardiol 2003; 15:380–384.

10

Controversy and Convergence

HAROLD L. DAUERMAN and
BURTON E. SOBEL

University of Vermont
Burlington, Vermont, U.S.A.

This book was written to develop a perspective, referred to as pharmacoinvasive therapy, and to present nomenclature designed to explicitly and logically define an overall approach for the treatment of patients with acute ST elevation myocardial infarction (STEMI). Previous terminology such as "facilitated angioplasty" has, we believe, obfuscated key concepts rather than articulated them in a fashion consistent with their value (1).

The early evolution of coronary thrombolysis and of primary balloon angioplasty for the treatment of STEMI led to an unfortunate dichotomy. What resulted from initial attempts to combine the two was a strict adherence by particular practitioners to either a pharmacological or mechanical approach rather than to one combining the two modalities. Subsequently, advances in the pharmacology of coronary thrombolysis and in percutaneous coronary intervention (PCI) set the stage for revisiting the possibility that combined therapy would be particularly beneficial. As pointed out in several chapters preceding this one, strict adherence to either a pharmacological or mechanical approach for treatment of STEMI entails inherent limitations that appear likely to be obviated by pharmacoinvasive therapy. The developments addressed in Chapters 1, 6, and 8 have rendered obsolete initial fears of combining pharmacological and mechanical approaches. In addition, they have supported the likelihood that prompt, pharmacologically induced recanalization and consolidation of benefit with PCI is an optimal strategy for treatment of many patients with STEMI.

Utilization of PCI after antecedent treatment with a fibrinolytic agent may entail risk not encountered with PCI alone and certainly does not simplify PCI. Thus, the term "facilitated PCI" is misleading. It implies that the purpose of antecedent fibrinolysis is to somehow simplify subsequent PCI or facilitate its performance. In fact, the objective of antecedent fibrinolysis is to diminish the duration of ischemia, accelerate initial recanalization, enhance salvage of myocardium as a result of the acceleration, and prolong the temporal window during which definitive recanalization achieved with subsequent PCI can be optimally effective. Advances in PCI involving the use of stents, distal embolic protection, and other sophisticated devices are not designed merely to simplify performance of the intervention. Instead, they are designed to enhance outcome. The same applies to pharmacoinvasive therapy.

In Chapters 2 and 4 the development of life-saving approaches for treatment of patients with STEMI is described. Initially explored in small, rigorously controlled studies, approaches developed were demonstrably beneficial with respect to biological and physiological endpoints. Subsequent multicenter, randomized clinical trials demonstrated benefit in terms of clinical outcome. Nevertheless, as so clearly stated in these elegantly written chapters, controversy persisted despite the performance of numerous, "definitive" large-scale trials. Much of the controversy reflected confounding influences, particularly advances over time that complicated planning, execution, and interpretation of results in such trials. Thus, whereas a pilot study of primary PCI or of coronary thrombolysis might have indicated benefit for a specifically defined population, planning of subsequent large-scale randomized clinical trials required some guesswork regarding the need to incorporate progress made following completion of the pilot study. For example, such progress may have pointed to altered dosing and timing of administration of anticoagulant and antiplatelet agents. Other potential alterations that might pertain would include the extent to which elderly patients should be included in the trial, the optimal timing of administration of drugs or performance of mechanical interventions, and the extent to which centers with relatively low numbers of procedures performed should be included. Because large-scale multicenter clinical trials inevitably require protracted intervals to plan, develop, perform, and complete, no matter how important or how clear the results from a given trial of a fibrinolytic agent or primary PCI may have been, advances in therapy pertinent to both will undoubtedly have evolved in the protracted interval during which the trial was performed. These considerations require regularly revisiting matters that may have appeared to have been settled by results in a particular "landmark" trial.

It may be the case that some concepts underlying therapy of STEMI are indeed timeless. It became clear from several early trials with diverse interventions that time to treatment was a pivotal determinant of the benefit that could be conferred by an intervention (2). This, in fact, underlies the concept of pharmacoinvasive therapy. The combination of a recanalization-implemented fibrinolytic drug coupled with subsequent PCI to consolidate recanalization offers a promise of synergistic benefits. Unfortunately, limitations in technology (balloon angioplasty) and pharmacology (aspirin, unfractionated heparin, and non-fibrin-selective fibrinolytic agents) undoubtedly influenced the results of early trials entailing combination therapy (3). Thus, interpretation of the early results obtained are, ironically, time limited. Subsequently, trials such as PACT, SPEED, and TIMI 10B/14B began to point toward safety with a pharmacoinvasive approach (4–6). Most recently the results in SIAM-3 and GRACIA-2 have lent additional impetus to the need to explore the potential benefit of pharmacoinvasive therapy in the treatment of STEMI (7,8).

As discussed in Chapters 7 and 9, one size does not fit all. The risk of stroke in elderly patients given fibrinolytic drugs must be addressed with respect to utilizing a pharmacoinvasive approach. Prompt, complete, and sustained recanalization and restoration of myocardial perfusion are imperative objectives in all patients with STEMI. Thus, the risk of stroke in the elderly must be addressed by refinement of treatment modalities in this particularly high-risk group. Such an approach is suggested in Chapter 7, in which Drs. Antman and Braunwald

Trial	N	Pharmacoinvasive	Primary PCI	Bleeding	Efficacy
CAPTIM	840	tPA/UFH 33% with urgent PCI	UFH	Equal	PIT best < 2 hrs
GRACIA-2	212	TNK/Enoxaparin 3–12 hrs to PCI	UFH or Abciximab	Equal (3%)	PIT better ST resolution; infarct size the same
SIAM-3	163	RPA/UFH PCI at 3.5 hours	RPA/UFH PCI at 2 weeks	10% for PIT; 7% for lytics	PIT superior to lytics alone
BRAVE	253	5U RPA + Abcixmab	Abciximab	6% for PIT 2% for Primary PCI	MACE and infarct size the same

MACE = major adverse coronary events, PIT = pharmacoinvasive therapy, RPA = reteplase, TNK = tenecteplase, tPA = tissue-type plasminogen activator, UFH = unfractionated heparin

Figure 10.1   Current trials of pharmacoinvasive therapy are small to moderate in size. They all employ stenting and fibrin-specific thrombolytic agents. One, CAPTIM, is a classic thrombolysis compared with primary PCI trial (12). However, a pharmacoinvasive approach emerges in the fibrinolytic treatment arm. The other three trials deal with safety and efficacy of the pharmacoinvasive approach. The ongoing ASSENT-4 trial will be the largest trial to date comparing pharmacoinvasive therapy with primary PCI.

propose a "rule of 75" as a point of departure. They propose that rather than forgoing the option of antecedent fibrinolysis preceding PCI in elderly patients with STEMI, a 25% reduction in the dose of the fibrinolytic agent and the doses of conjunctive agents such as low molecular weight heparin is merited and should be tested rigorously in a clinical trial. Until this approach or an analogous one has been demonstrated to provide the necessary safety, treatment of high-risk elderly patients with STEMI with a pharmacoinvasive approach will remain controversial (9).

Fortuitously, trials incorporating pharmacoinvasive therapy are proceeding (Fig. 10.1). Among them, several such as BRAVE, GRACIA-2, and SIAM-3 are focusing on the safety and efficacy of early PCI following antecedent fibrinolysis (7,8,10). The safety of the

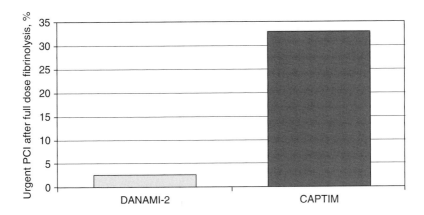

Figure 10.2   The emergence of pharmacoinvasive therapy in practice is evident by comparing the approaches actually used in CAPTIM and DANAMI-2 (11,12). There was >10-fold difference in the use of urgent PCI after full-dose thrombolytics in CAPTIM compared with the earlier DANAMI-2 trial. Favorable results in CAPTIM's fibrinolytic arm may be directly related to the high use of early PCI subsequently.

approach appears to be remarkably different from that described when coronary thrombolysis and balloon angioplasty were first combined more than 20 years ago. Although limitations of the trials completed to date and of ASSENT-4 are well described in Chapter 8, an interesting phenomenon is obviously occurring. If one compares results in CAPTIM and DANAMI-2, a striking difference is apparent (11,12). In CAPTIM, 33% of patients treated with fibrinolytic agents in the prehospital phase underwent early PCI. By contrast, in the earlier DANAMI-1 trial, only 2.5% of those randomized to fibrinolysis subsequently underwent urgent PCI (Fig. 10.2). As judged from this difference, the concept of early implementation of PCI after antecedent treatment with a fibrinolytic agent is becoming more attractive in the care of patients with STEMI, even in trials that are not formally investigating pharmacoinvasive therapy.

The remarkable improvement in survival of patients with STEMI over the past 3 decades (13) reflects bold initiatives and advances in technology and pharmacology. Experience with both coronary thrombolysis and primary PCI demonstrates unequivocally that recanalization of the infarct-related artery is life-saving. Results with both modalities support the view that minimization of the interval between the onset of ischemia and the initiation of reperfusion is a pivotal determinant of benefit. Results with both modalities demonstrate that persistence and completeness of recanalization are pivotal as well (14–16). Thus, the concept that early, complete, and sustained recanalization of the infarct-related artery and restoration of myocardial perfusion is the penultimate objective of initial treatment of patients with STEMI has been well substantiated. Pharmacoinvasive therapy offers particular promise in achieving this objective.

REFERENCES

1. Dauerman HL, Sobel BE. Synergistic treatment of ST-segment elevation myocardial infarction with pharmacoinvasive recanalization. *J Am Coll Cardiol.* 2003;42:646-651.

2. Cannon CP, Gibson CM, Lambrew CT, et al. Relationship of symptom-onset-to-balloon time and door-to-balloon time with mortality in patients undergoing angioplasty for acute myocardial infarction. *JAMA.* 2000;283:2941-2947.

3. Comparison of invasive and conservative strategies after treatment with intravenous tissue plasminogen activator in acute myocardial infarction. Results of the thrombolysis in myocardial infarction (TIMI) phase II trial. The TIMI Study Group. *N Engl J Med.* 1989;320:618-627.

4. Herrmann HC, Moliterno DJ, Ohman EM, et al. Facilitation of early percutaneous coronary intervention after reteplase with or without abciximab in acute myocardial infarction: results from the SPEED (GUSTO-4 Pilot) Trial. *J Am Coll Cardiol.* 2000;36:1489-1496.

5. Ross AM, Coyne KS, Reiner JS, et al. A randomized trial comparing primary angioplasty with a strategy of short-acting thrombolysis and immediate planned rescue angioplasty in acute myocardial infarction: the PACT trial. PACT investigators. Plasminogen-activator Angioplasty Compatibility Trial. *J Am Coll Cardiol.* 1999;34:1954-1962.

6. Schweiger MJ, Cannon CP, Murphy SA, et al. Early coronary intervention following pharmacological therapy for acute myocardial infarction (the combined TIMI 10B–TIMI 14 experience). *Am J Cardiol.* 2001;88:831-836.

7. O'Neill WW, Dixon SR. The year in interventional cardiology. *J Am Coll Cardiol.* 2004;43:875-890.

8. Scheller B, Hennen B, Hammer B, et al. Beneficial effects of immediate stenting after thrombolysis in acute myocardial infarction. *J Am Coll Cardiol.* 2003;42:634-641.

9. Thiemann DR. Primary angioplasty for elderly patients with myocardial infarction: theory, practice and possibilities. *J Am Coll Cardiol.* 2002;39:1729-1732.

10. Kastrati A, Mehilli J, Schlotterbeck K, et al. Early administration of reteplase plus abciximab vs. abciximab alone in patients with acute myocardial infarction referred for percutaneous coronary intervention: a randomized controlled trial. *JAMA.* 2004;291:947-954.

11. Andersen HR, Nielsen TT, Rasmussen K, et al. A comparison of coronary angioplasty with fibrinolytic therapy in acute myocardial infarction. *N Engl J Med.* 2003;349:733-742.

12. Bonnefoy E, Lapostolle F, Leizorovicz A, et al. Primary angioplasty versus prehospital fibrinolysis in acute myocardial infarction: a randomised study. *Lancet.* 2002;360:825-829.

13. Furman MI, Dauerman HL, Goldberg RJ, et al. Twenty-two year (1975 to 1997) trends in the incidence, in-hospital and long-term case fatality rates from initial Q-wave and non-Q-wave myocardial infarction: a multi-hospital, community-wide perspective. *J Am Coll Cardiol.* 2001; 37:1571-1580.

14. Gibson CM, Karha J, Murphy SA, et al. Early and long-term clinical outcomes associated with reinfarction following fibrinolytic administration in the Thrombolysis in Myocardial Infarction trials. *J Am Coll Cardiol.* 2003;42:7-16.

15. Gibson CM, Cannon CP, Murphy SA, et al. Relationship of the TIMI myocardial perfusion grades, flow grades, frame count, and percutaneous coronary intervention to long-term outcomes after thrombolytic

administration in acute myocardial infarction. *Circulation.* 2002;105: 1909-1913.

16. Gibson CM, Cannon CP, Murphy SA, et al. Relationship of TIMI myocardial perfusion grade to mortality after administration of thrombolytic drugs. *Circulation.* 2000;101:125-130.

Index